I0693357

Fat, Fifty, and Finished

Where Are You Now?

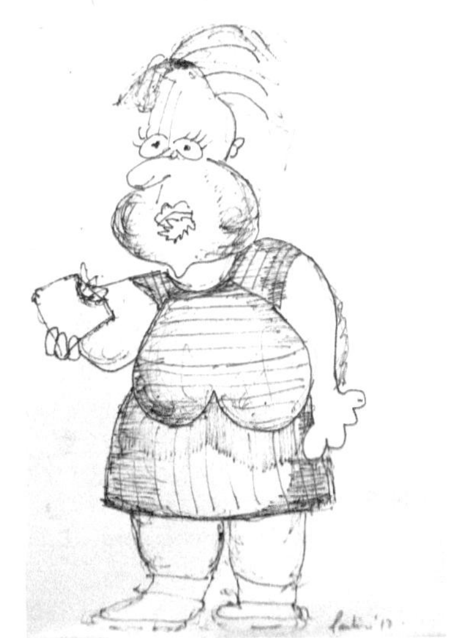

Caroline Pledger

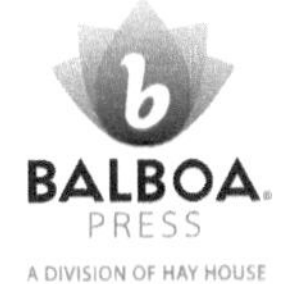

BALBOA
PRESS

A DIVISION OF HAY HOUSE

Balboa Press books may be ordered through booksellers or by contacting:

Balboa Press
A Division of Hay House
1663 Liberty Drive
Bloomington, IN 47403
www.balboapress.com
1 (877) 407-4847

Because of the dynamic nature of the Internet, any web addresses or links contained in this book may have changed since publication and may no longer be valid. The views expressed in this work are solely those of the author and do not necessarily reflect the views of the publisher, and the publisher hereby disclaims any responsibility for them.

The author of this book does not dispense medical advice or prescribe the use of any technique as a form of treatment for physical, emotional, or medical problems without the advice of a physician, either directly or indirectly. The intent of the author is only to offer information of a general nature to help you in your quest for emotional and spiritual well-being. In the event you use any of the information in this book for yourself, which is your constitutional right, the author and the publisher assume no responsibility for your actions.

Any people depicted in imagery supplied by Caroline Pledger are models and such images are being used for illustrative purposes only. All illustrations are the work of Illustrator, Author Photographer, Caroline Pledger and are owned by copyright Caroline Pledger

Print information available on the last page.

ISBN: 978-1-9822-0018-3 (sc)
ISBN: 978-1-9822-0020-6 (hc)
ISBN: 978-1-9822-0019-0 (e)

Library of Congress Control Number: 2018903275

Balboa Press rev. date: 04/18/2018

CONTENTS

Introduction

Fat, fifty & finished… where are you now?! is a social commentary regarding all aspects of health and how each component works in unison to create wellbeing and prosperity. It encompasses the idea that you are the *one* that is truly responsible for your own health and wellbeing. Despite where you may be on the disease continuum, and regardless of age, you have the ability to intervene, to reverse and to regenerate to produce a sense of vitality. Although my intention is honourable and for the good of all beings, it is somewhat (or at least I have been told), as subtle as a sledge hammer to remind ourselves that there is personal accountability regarding health and your own perception of health. Health begins in the library of the mind and is affected by our internal physiology and our external environment. Perhaps a rehash of old news but it is much easier to check-up with yourself now and again, so you don't fall into the abyss of declining health and disease!

This book is dedicated to anyone who is interested in maintaining a quality of life regardless of age and bears relevance to the holistic model of health to achieve that. This book is also a wakeup call to urge us to become more aware and accountable for our declining health, especially as we age. It is not designed to infuriate or attack you in any way shape or form. But the fact that you may feel uncomfortable whilst reading it means that I have touched upon a raw nerve in some Instances.

After all you are responsible for you. As egocentric as that may sound, your life really is and will always be about you!

A long time ago, in my teenage years, a dear friend of mine gave this poem to me. It has never left my memory, moving me forward in the lowest of lows, encouraging me to believe that ultimately your thoughts can make it so and ultimately, you are responsible for you!

The man who wins is the man who thinks he can

If you think you are beaten, you are
If you think you dare not, you don't,
If you like to win, but think you can't
It is almost certain that you won't.
If you think you will lose, you're lost,
For out of the world you'll find
Success begins with a fellow's will,
It's all in the state of mind.
If you think you are outclassed, you are,
You've got to think high to rise.
You've got to be sure of yourself before you ever win a prize.
Life's battles don't always go to the stronger and faster man,
But soon or late, the man who wins is the man who thinks he can!
Walter D Wintle

1

—∽—

THE MONSTER WITHIN

The vision that you glorify in your mind, the ideal that you enthrone in your heart, this, you will build your life by, and this, you will become.

—James Allen

Champions are created, not born. It is you who becomes the champion, the light, or the monster—the darkness of your own life, the creator of your destiny, the creator of your life. The commitment words, "In sickness or in health," uttered in the marriage ceremony should be the words spoken to yourself throughout your whole life, as life is ultimately related to the comfort or the discomfort of being. You must live with yourself and your thoughts, buzzing around your head like the white noise of a 1960s TV set, the idle chitter-chatter of nonsense that can make or, alternatively, break you. Your life is about seven inches—the length from ear to ear. This is where your life begins—or ends! A diagnosis of mental illness, autoimmune disease, diabetes, or cancer may be likened to paraplegia—something deemed as a negative in your life that can somehow be turned into a positive. Doctors may tell you that you will never walk again; yet you defy those odds and not only walk but run a marathon! So how can the forever wheelchair-bound paraplegic overcome this disability? How does it happen? Are our lives measured by and based on authoritative opinion or the confinements of the limiting beliefs within our own mind-sets?

Harsh words, but true. The truth is that you design your life, beginning with a thought that dictates your actions. When do we ever consider our own actions as major contributors to acquiring any disease? Are we predisposed to becoming unhealthy, or do we create the environment to disarm our health? Why is it that a person who has chosen to live healthily—whatever that means—for twenty years is suddenly diagnosed with pancreatic cancer at the age of sixty-five, or a man who has just turned fifty suddenly gets brain cancer? Everyone has a past and everyone has a different perception of health. For all we know, a person suddenly confronted with a life-threatening illness could have been a chronic cocaine addict or a raving sex addict at fifteen and acquired an STD or, in the free-for-all, loving '60s acquired hepatitis B or been an alcoholic and suffered chronic liver disease for years. Who is to know the real cause of disease? There's an old saying that goes something like this "what is whispered in secret someday will be shouted from the roof top'. To be sure, sooner or later, in some shape or form, your life will catch up with you—karma's a bitch!

Extreme behaviours, addictions, and over-the-top fads may lead to a *What the—?* moment and suddenly the question *Why me?* It's a bit like overnight fame. Fame, like a chronic disease, comes not by luck but a combination of long years of hard work and only looks like it happened over night!

The iron fist in the velvet glove, Margaret Thatcher, one of the longest-serving prime ministers in the history of British politics, sums up the concept in this statement: "Be careful of your thoughts because they become your words, be careful about your words because they become your actions and be careful about your actions because they become your habits and be careful about your habits, as they then will determine your character." Einstein also said, "For every action there is an equal and or opposite reaction." Assuming, that this is so, whatever we do daily will dictate the circumstances of our lives and, predictably, the outcome of our health. This is where our daily habits, either good or bad, matter. You know that if you continually eat biscuits, you will eventually put on weight. You know that if you have too much alcohol, you will wake up with a raging hangover. You know if you take medication there will be an action or an opposing reaction. You know this because you have done it or somebody else has done it before you! On your part, this is your responsibility. Once you understand this simple concept, claim this knowledge, and accept your actions as your own, you take ownership and therefore accept accountability. In other words, you become responsible for **you**, your life, and your health. I guess it starts with *accountability, acceptance and an attitude.*

A true champion has a foundation of values and convictions. Champions go out on a limb and tread a different path than most. Champions know what they want, know who they are, and understand what they need to do to be one! Artists, politicians, athletes, bodybuilders, and marathon runners are often deemed as champions espousing to live to the standards they have set for themselves. Whilst they may be extreme, they truly appreciate the difficulties and obstacles of becoming one. They have learnt to become their one life hero! The heroes of our time, like our great leaders, are not always liked but are well respected for staying true to themselves. These champions recognise hardships delete the word excuses from their lives and dare to play out their lives differently, running the gauntlet of being heralded as mad, sad, or lost. Other champions don't accept their fate but change their circumstances to match their true values. For others being a champion may be just getting out of bed each day! None the less being a champion doesn't necessarily mean winning or losing but being aware and upholding positive attributes that contribute to your life and ultimately your overall health.

Like any young girl getting into trouble, I was punished accordingly with either a smack or a lecture. As I sat in a corner sulking, my father would remind me that I had no one else to blame but myself. As much as I hated to admit it—he was right. He was also big on the word attitude and it may be our attitude to a multitude of everyday occurrences that invariably influences our actions. Your thoughts and actions create the problems in your life. Your mind becomes irrevocably married to the problem, the disaster, the disorder, and then, ultimately, the disease. It is you who marries the white noise of buzzing thoughts that pervade your mind. We all have that monster within, and our thoughts provide the energy that yields an outcome. If only we could acknowledge this as a basic truth, then we could fully understand that we too, can alter the scenarios of our lives and ultimately our health and well-being.

You may remember a brilliant courtroom scene in the movie *A Few Good Men*. Jack Nicholson's character, a stoic, medal-adorned officer in the US Navy, blurts out aggressively, "You want the truth." He goes on in an irritated manner, "You can't handle the truth!" This book is about understanding that you play a huge part in your own existence and are thereby responsible for your own health—in other words, the truth. When someone tells us the truth, most of us don't *really* want to listen, for many reasons. We may be come defensive as someone may have threatened our way of being. We may become dismissive and live in denial, as we hand over the control of our lives to others in hope that a situation may disperse or simply disappear. In other words, we give away our power. Most of us treat our health like that. Having pertinent and up-to-date information regarding health and well-being, gives you the know-how. Knowledge is power, but if you don't know what you don't know, how can you know what you don't know? And knowledge is power only when you practice what you know. True knowledge is action. To know what you now know is to grow; this is true power. Surprising as it is, most people spend more time planning their holidays or weddings than taking care of their health, and yet without your health, there can be no wealth! It's a rather rhetorical question, but what are your values, and are you really living in accordance with those?

Is Your Health Part of Your Values?

> You are your choices.
>
> —Jean Paul Satre

According to the World Health organization (WHO), health is a "state of complete physical mental and social wellbeing, rather than merely the absence of disease or infirmity." Understanding how nutrition attenuates the disease continuum is only one aspect of truly recognizing health within a holistic framework. It is also looking at the person, not merely on a physical level but within the context of prosperity of all aspects of health. Nutrition is the fundamental foundation to health on all levels and in a medical world, the one aspect that we have overlooked. Only now do we recognize nutrition as important in determining our health status and, ultimately, our lives.

Your genetic blueprint does not make you fat or give rise to hormonal problems, depression, eating disorders, ADHD, or bipolar disorder, or cancer—need I go on? But, sometimes and too often, it serves as an excuse for not getting on and creating the life that we desire or were born to lead. Too many people marry their disorders and create their lives around them, accepting that this is the way it is. Over many years of observing and struggling personally with the question of why we become so sick, I've figured that unnecessary thoughts like worry, fear, and the threat of the unknown just make things worse. Ultimately, we are feeding the energy of fear, omitting gratitude for the here and now. Therefore, creating

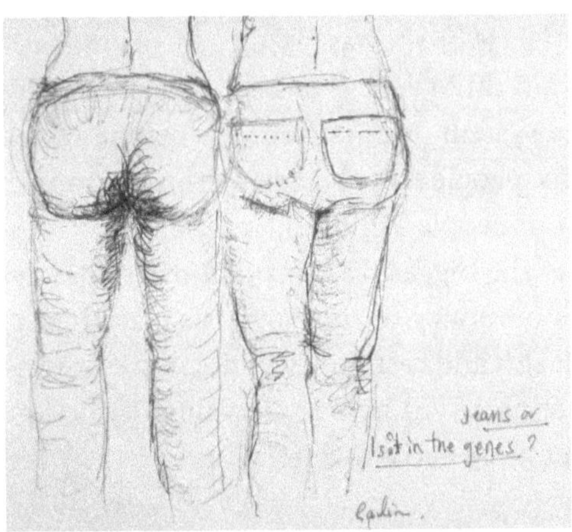

more of what we are afraid of. To get a little personal, recently I was asked why I was not as successful as I should have been. The concept of success is subjective and can be translated to mean various independent benchmarks. At that time, I knew that he had referred to money as a yardstick for success. I thought about this for a while and responded, "from a lack of confidence and self-belief. Predominantly fear". My mind meandered over the past 12 years since my divorce. I had been dancing with disease for most part of my life, but since my marriage breakdown I was merely surviving, yet alone living. With no doubt this has been ultimately my creation as instead of coming up with a solution, I was too busy focusing on the problem. I was also going through menopause which changed the goal posts significantly. But the one thing that has become obvious is that by altering your biochemistry, through nutrition and oxygenation has a colossal effect on your body, your wellbeing and your life.

Obviously, my value on money has been less with more value placed on my health. The question is how much value do you place on your health and are we doing anything to preserve your own? Value systems are important guidelines to keep you in check to be who you are. For example, if you stroll into a meeting four minutes late the person conducting the meeting maybe infuriated by your lack of attention to punctuality and respect. It may not seem important to you but to the other person, his or her reaction indicates that it obviously is. He or she has placed a lot of emphasis on being punctual and anything less is not good enough. It's part of the existing value system. Money, too can be one of the highest priorities in many people's lives and for this reason we see an exorbitant amount of people killing themselves (or others) to reach their goal. One of the biggest reasons that marriages are breaking down is the lack of money or the emphasis placed on it. Money cannot buy your health and certainly will not make you any less vulnerable to contracting any illness or unwanted affliction. Perhaps _we need_ to be a bit more accountable!

"Do not follow where the path may lead. Go instead, where there is no path and leave a trail".

Ralph waldo Emerson

It is highly probable that by not being clearly conscious we have created the problems and the challenges within various aspects of our life. If we look realistically at our own actions and their ramifications, we can either make changes or accept the consequences. Let's not pretend though that they don't exist or that <u>it</u> won't happen to you. Accepting this reality, by living in the moment and being present, we can appreciate life as a gift, not one to be endured. It doesn't have to be a struggle. It doesn't have to be doom and gloom. It doesn't have to be complicated, or, as we gasp for our last breath, whisper the words "thank god that's over". We are the managers of our own lives and consequently we do have a say.

Life, disease and our health is simply all about management. Like diabetes, obesity, mental health and cancer (at an early stage) are disorders which can be regulated by managing all areas of our lives. Like all illnesses, they have the potential to become a persistent part of you, dormant or activated. You have the power to choose the path to wellness or allow an illness to take over your life with strength and tenacity that overwhelms you, like a living being. A monster within that crosses over to the dark. Given certain conditions which enable this to happen, the monster can then become your master. Let's make choices, free of illusions, as maintaining illusions, wishes and living in denial, can be hazardous to your health!

<u>Today is tomorrows history.</u>

In a world where we look to medical intervention to control our health issues, health has escalated out of proportion. We are failing to meaningfully reform the way health care is approached. Why are we not closer to finding a cure for any disease or ailment in a tablet, supplement or a pharmaceutical? Why, in our modern-day world, too many of us are afflicted with disease or disorder? Has disease become a word that is synonymous with economic expansion and modern-day living? One in **four** people in the world will be affected by mental or neurological disorders at some point in their lives. Around 450 million people currently suffer from such conditions, placing mental disorders among the leading causes of ill-health and disability worldwide. (1) In the United States alone over 700 billion dollars is spent on dementia annually whilst approximately 300 billion is spent on cancer yet we fear this disease more than the other. Once upon a time the odds of getting cancer was one in twenty but now it is one in two. Having these unfavourable odds, the likelihood is that at one point or another in our, sophisticated, technologically and medically advanced world it is likely that we could end up with that disease. The real question we should be asking ourselves, as we take the pokie pilgrimage on a Sunday evening is not how we want to live life but how do we want to leave this life?

I, We have looked to the past and historically the treatment of disease has been varied. Those with new and different ideas often face fierce opposition by the medical establishment and government bureaucracies. History is dotted with new concepts that have faced opposition for fear of them that sit outside the internal establishment may actually be right. In 1872, even Louis Pasteur's '*Theory of Germs*', was pronounced a "ridiculous fiction" by a Pierre Pachet, Professor of physiology.(2) When it comes to emergency interventions modern medicine is still the best in the world, but when it comes to disorders or major diseases like chronic illness this approach has failed as Modern industrial medicine is designed to <u>treat disease with medication or surgery.</u> (3) The focus is on treating the symptoms and not the cause, ignoring the interrelationships between the physical, mental and psychosocial criteria of health. Before the twentieth century, in European, Indian and Chinese cultures, medicinal foods and herbs were used with a great deal of success treating the cause and symptoms of diseases. Today this is called Functional Medicine.

Functional medicine aims to rebalance the body from disorder to order and from disease to ease. Advancement does not always serve for the advantage of society and diverse ways of dealing with old problems have been denounced, which is clearly where we are going wrong.

In our Advancing world, Modern Medicine has looked at curing chronic and debilitating disease by utilising medicines that have been tried and tested on human guinea pigs for decades. Newspapers and the media announce that a new drug has been found from clinical trials. Whilst proven to be effective on rodents, these stories forget to mention that more deaths are found on real humans than recorded, because of these drugs. Traditional medical dogma leads us to believe "this is the way it is, so therefore it should be" and most of us accept this. Society, our beliefs or lack thereof and a call to survive this physical world dictates a response of instant gratification, hence the search for a single bullet or one drug which will fix all scenarios. It seems illogical to try to regulate physiology with a chemical to expect a positive biological result. Both pharmaceutical and nutraceutical companies compete and race head to head, to cash in on what's hot and current. They both can be blamed for providing band aids to symptoms and bypassing the root cause. In a world hell bent on surviving, maintaining symptoms and looking for a quick fix, the commercial model keeps everybody fed!

Personal experience has provided me with my fair share of traditional medical intervention. Having spent time in an institution for having anorexia and labelled with many mental health disorders I have grappled with this perspective of treatment. Near starving myself to death, obviously becoming nutritiously deficient I nearly reached the point of no return. The worst part of such a disease is that you do not even realise that you are ill, you just think you are fat!!! From years of battling, cursing the Doctors, screaming fits, histrionic outbursts and living on struggle street, l have learned to live with them. Manage it. For the most part, it is up to you. Don't worry, there have been times when I have wished for a frontal lobotomy to correct the mental challenges that can be overwhelming to the point where you sit on the precipice of falling off the edge of the world. It must be, all about management, making the decision to be well and committing to survive and live to your full potential. Unfortunate, but true, we must take some form of accountability when it comes to our health and for most of us, we don't get out of our own way or maybe we just don't care, or worse can't be bothered! If nothing changes, nothing will change! Famous last words, I know.

When a strange mole appeared on my décolletage, I did not hesitate to use the infamous and illegal black salve to the shock of my doctor. A little white image of a crab appears on my chest as a reminder to check my progress on a health basis. This was, by far a better option than going under the knife and risking it not being "all cut out". I decided that I would implement the ketogenic diet and trained almost every day convinced that I could deplete the energy from my body, so I could live to tell another tale. Six weeks later whilst running the gold Coast marathon, someone asked what my motivation was. I mean to say, who would run their first marathon at the ripe age of forty-six? I answered as smoothly as possible, whilst settling into a nice rhythm and pace, "cancer"! I finished that race, just over the 4-hour mark. Perhaps my ambition was greater than my ability, but I had a great foundation of health and a lot of 'miles' in the legs. Whilst I was secretly a little disappointed, I had to be happy with that. Another tick off my bucket list.

Several times I followed the instructions from my general practitioner and several gynaecologists by having invasive exploration for endometrial cancer. Endothelial hyperplasia in a non-reproducing female in her 50s is not uncommon, however there were other symptoms that matched this type of cancer profile. Even so, whilst a precautionary measure to check for a malignancy. It was actually a pro-inflammatory exercise on both a physical and emotional level exacerbating anxiety and thoughts of what if, and for what. Their solution even before we had one, was to implant a Merina (a uterine device) or what I call a UFO an (unidentified flaming object) to alter my reproductive hormones. To hell with that! I had some knowledge of this "Merina" and the detrimental effects on so many women under my care. Already living with hormonal hysteria, I was not about to opt for more! I asked the question why and It's hardly surprising my reaction was quite defensive. Even being slightly sedated, the poor man had to duck and weave from the wrath that blurted from my unyielding tongue! You are going to put what where???? Not in this life time. It was a situation where I felt pressured by others to do what they wanted me to do. Having a great relationship with my GP, he had already suggested previously, to get rid of it, meaning a hysterectomy. "After all," he said candidly, "it had done its job". I sat and thought quietly for a few minutes then looked up at him and said very coolly, "have you ever considered having your penis cut off?". We didn't talk much about any further options after that, I don't know why. However, a surgeon is designed to cut, operate remove and eliminate. It is his job, a way of keeping food on the table! Precautionary tests? invasive surgery? Another counsellor? Seek and you shall find and then what? Another pill? An implant? A removal of an important functioning part of your body? Is this our only option? What ever happened to BP? (Before pills) It's a bit like smart phones…… what on earth did we do before them?

I urge anyone that has been told you have a 'predisposition' or have an 'existing disorder' and is prescribed a pharmaceutical to ask why. Why do I have high cholesterol? Why do I have hypertension? Why do I have hormonal dysfunction? Why am I depressed? It seems common place that medicine of this nature is being prescribed without addressing the 'Whys' and not the question how Can I overcome the disorder before taking a drug? I see far too many people that consume a handful of tablets every day, yet do not actually know what they are and why they are having them. I urge you to become the critical enquirer and get to the heart of the real problem.

The concept of the disease continuum.

Most people love to talk about themselves. In fact, most people love to talk about their condition or their health problem. It starts when we are young, the sore on our knee, a pretended cough that keeps us home from school. Or the headaches that provide a scape goat for not going to dinner with the out-laws! As a writer that visits local cafes, I overhear many conversations about "health". For most part of the discussion, we talk about our problems, the Doctor, the specialist and the problem. Not once is there any correlation between themselves or their responsibility in this scenario. Old people always talk about their hearts and their bowels over having their cup of chinos!!! Great coffee conversation, yet as boring as this sounds this seems to be the way it is.

The way most of us think often misses the correlation between the basic biochemical processes, order of inter-related systems, human psychic and the physical embodiment of any disease. The traditional medical model is not necessarily focused on this and for this very reason, misguided. It misses one of the most fundamental laws of physiology, biology and disease; *the continuum concept*. This concept begins with optimal health usually at birth then moving through to hidden imbalances, dysfunction, disorders, disease and finally death. The four ds of life. Anywhere along that continuum, from the cradle to the grave we can intervene and reverse the process by focusing on living and loving and not the conflicting solution on offer, such as fighting or killing! It is unfortunate the conventional treatments that a sick person must choose from, is in fact more harmful long term than the disease itself. If the quality of life is compromised over the quantity of a life filled with vile debilitating side effects that merely sustains breath in our body, then what's the point????? Is this merely surviving and ambling clumsily through the motions of life? Is this control or management? Is this really living?

Improving your health is a very empowering experience. It's like stacking the dominos. Improving this compartment will reward you with a powerful overflow effect on the rest of your life. To take a step away from current dogma about conventional medicine is brave. To deny consumerism, popular fads and defy current medical and traditional dogma takes courage and education. There is enormous amount of contradictory opinion between holistic-nutritional-naturopathic practitioners and medical ideology. As the majority of the latter eliminates the obvious and does not accept or understand the connection between diet and other aspects of health underpinning the course of chronic disease.

My question to you is "can you make a positive contribution to your own life to make a difference?" It is my hope that my creativity and sharing of knowledge, provides an insight to why we have become sick in the first place and to point out the dangers of our modern day life in contributing to disease. If this alters only one person's life, then that is better than not doing anything at all! If we can contribute to creating a world where we want to live in, instead of complaining, shifting blame and worrying about the world as it is. Altruistic, I know but living half asleep, wandering around this planet like half dead corpses, trying to fit in with what someone else has proposed that life should be, is killing us. Our own life is slowly killing us. Our jobs are killing us. Stress is killing us, over indulgence and keeping up with the Jones's (whoever the jones is) are all slowly killing us. By the time you reach midpoint of your life and find your loose breasts swaying in the breeze, your derriere following you like a swollen shadow, you then begin to think, is this it and perhaps what now?

Everything costs. We live in a physical world with primary needs for survival like shelter, food and water, everything else is secondary. There is unnecessary emphasis placed on what is deemed important in our society. The more we understand the fundamentals of our life and our health and omit the unnecessary the less broken or scarred we will be. "Only actions turn knowledge into wisdom" (anonymous). People often ask me, what or how can I change? Most people already know the answer, but what they are really asking is … What is the easiest way? The solutions are simple, being conscious, fully engaged, becoming aware, taking time to be responsible for you and being mindful that you have the power to manage you, before you get to that fat, fifty and finished state. You can make a difference to your world and it has to start with you and it has to start today.

Your life …… your world, and in the words of the Thai people …………… up to you!

2

THE ULTIMATE DISEASE - .... CANCER.

When I first heard of cancer, it was not the disease as such but in the context of the astrological zodiac signs. A constellation of stars and when the word translates from Latin to English it means "crab". Ironically, the zodiac sign of cancer associates with the image of the crab. The idea of cancer and the crab inter-twined in around 500 BC when Hippocrates, the Greek father of Modern medicine, incised the surface of a breast cancer of a Persian Princess. He described the foreign body as "carcinos", meaning swollen crab. In other words, it looked like an inflamed crab with a larger body than his head and legs that were stretched outwards. He then coined the word "carcinoma" and later, Celsus translated carcinoma into Latin to the word "cancer", and this became the name we unfortunately, know only too well.

In evolution of all disease where there is no dispute from experts in their field, the origin of all disease is within the cell. (3) The cell is the basic and fundamental unit of life and as precious as life is, we know that there can be alterations to the cells life span. The protection of the cell is paramount to health more so as a babe and as we age beyond the midpoint in our life. Whilst cancer and other diseases can be genetically inherited other methods of spawning disease may be from either a bacterium, helicobacter pylori (stomach cancer), a virus like papilloma virus (cervical cancer), Epstein bar (lymphoma) and smoking (lung cancer). Yet diet and lifestyle stressors give rise to so many different cancers and are dominating as being a major cause. It is not only the internal environment but our external world that disturbs the balance or homeostasis of our finely tuned body.

In the framework of order there is chaos, yet harmonious at the same time. The body is continually and autonomously breaking down, repairing and rebuilding. A disruption of the normal process of cellular evolution can occur before and during our lives. Even whilst an embryo is developing, the nutritional status and the environment in which the mother lives has a profound effect on the health status quo of her infant. One of the most ancient of all diseases that alters or dysregulates the normal growth and development of a single cell is, Cancer. It is the disease that we want to avoid at all cost, Yet disorders not nipped in the bud could potentiate this disease ; prevention is way better than cure. You just don't want to go there! Yet we all have cancer and really it is a part of us.

When you are born, you have no say in what family you are born into and the DNA you are inheritably blessed with. The event of witnessing a birth of a new creature into this foreign world is beyond majestical. It is beyond any technological advancement and one of the most natural yet extraordinary events on this planet. The idea that a sperm and an ovum have kissed and joined together to create another life from one cell to create 206 different cells that form and create different tissues, organs and systems functioning in a harmonious union is beyond our imagination. Although explained by science it is still one of life's glorious joyous mysteries!

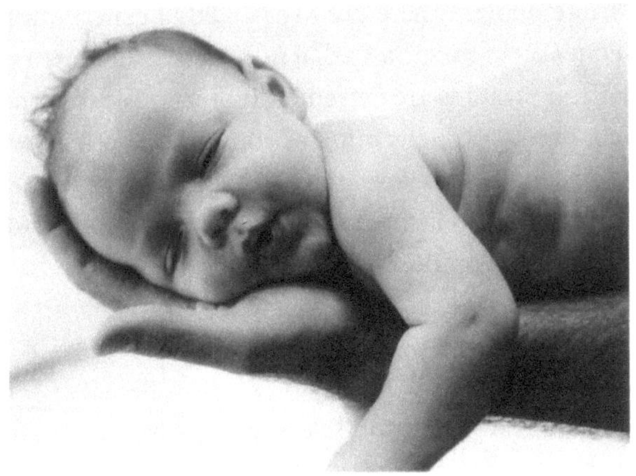

Your genetic material, good or bad has been passed on to you by your parents and from their parents. However, this does not mean that you should inherit Uncle Tom's wart on his nose or aunt Margie's sticking out ears or illness etc. Just because you have a genetic pre-disposition or a "mutant gene" for any disorder including mental disease, thyroid issues, obesity and cancer does not necessarily mean that **_you will get it!_** This is where epigenetics is at play. Taking precautionary measures and by being aware of what you firstly put into your mouth, and managing your environment, is part of a strategy to avoid such dis-ease. I mean, dis-ease is just your body not being at ease! Easier said than done … But hold on, I will explain.

A new born infant is purity and innocence with only the markings of both parent's DNA, from a physical point of view. DNA is the instructions to direct activities within the cell. This DNA is a long sequence of data that is unique to each individual, whilst borrowing a genetic sequence from our parents or even grandparents. There are 4 fundamental bases, from approximately 3 billion nucleotide bases, however it is the sequence of the order of the bases that determine our life's instructions. The black sheep of the family is probably just that, different from the herd, but yet, one of the same family.

To complicate matters there are over 20,0000 genes. These are the specific sequences of these bases that provide instruction to synthesise proteins. These proteins are extremely important as they may trigger a biological event and determine actions and inactivity within the body. Life circumstance cause genes to be silenced or expressed over time meaning they can be turned on (active) or turned off (dormant). This is epigenetics. In other words, it is a biological mechanism that switches genes on and off and epigenetics is at work all around us without our knowledge, day in and day out.

From what you eat, where you live and to whom you interact with, when you sleep, how you exercise and how you age are external modifications that do not change the DNA sequence, but instead, affect how cells "read" genes. In other words, you can shift or manoeuvre your genetic predisposition!! Quite A few years ago, a Hollywood star, had a faulty gene associated with breast cancer and decided to have a double mastectomy. Not an uncommon occurrence given the circumstance. A history of familial Breast cancer increased her expectation of a diagnosis. Having this operation is not necessarily a failsafe measure against the acquisition of cancer or any other such disease, however in her mind and according to specialists she took further precautionary measures to outwit this faulty gene by having another invasive surgery, a full hysterectomy. These operations are only a prophylactic as epigenetics as in what you do daily and your inner and outer environment will definitely define a disease's origin. Meaning that it is not always the faulty gene at play but a host of other factors really.

Our environment plays a huge role in disturbing our body's equilibrium and give rise to provide host for any disease including cancer. With ingestion of poisons, toxic foods, alcohol, cigarettes and lifestyle stresses we create an environment in which any disease can grow and flourish. Even going under a surgeon's knife to "cut bits out of your body", like a removal of tonsils, adenoids, gall bladder and appendix may not eliminate the original symptoms yet create inflammation perpetuating another cycle of inflammation. Those little bits of tissue and organs are conjunctions to other organs interconnecting with each other and are put there for a reason. The Adenoids, tonsils and appendix are a part of our immune system and without these your immune system may go into overdrive and eventually wear out. Your number one defence mechanism in your body, is your immune system and without it, disorders and eventually disease like a wild animal will thrive in an inflamed and weakened state.

The good thing about our bodies is that our Cells are constantly living and dying. There is one certainty in life and that life forces are continually changing. Given the fact that epigenetics can modify genes, you, therefore can manipulate circumstance to create ultimately the person and the life that you want. With this life, you can have both an improved physical and mental outlook. You do the best with what you have been given without giving into the fact that you have a faulty gene. Too many people use this as their excuse for their illnesses and succumb to relying on a system that provides medication that will eventually do more harm than good. Our filtration organs, in particular, the liver and the kidneys, ultimately end up with the sewerage and the difficult task of sorting, processing and dumping excess waste so that the system does not get bogged down! Pardon the pun!

On a cellular level the body can build and replace and even reshape every 7 years. Through this cycle of death and renewal you can restore the health of your cells. This encompasses the physical, mental, emotional and spiritual attributes of your body. We can renew healthy cells, through aiding the natural process of the body's ability to build, heal and to remove any unwanted and unnecessary cells. If we fully understand this, then *You have power and you have choice*. Your world is influenced by epigenetics meaning that you have the power to either turn yourself off, or rather turn yourself on!

This concept, in disease progression has been overlooked in modern medicine and this is where functional medicine intervenes. You see generally we are all focused on balance. We are all out of balance including nature, the world and the universe. We strive to fit in accordingly and end up failing miserably. The fact that the world is spinning out of control means that we need to rebalance to fit in with it. Too much emphasis is placed on what we think and how we feel and what we think we need to survive this forever changing world of ours, to the point that it is overwhelming furthering stress which is the very thing we need to avoid in the first place. Eat or be eaten! To function we need not only survive but to adapt to the conditions surrounding us. It is like adapting and evolving with the changes that occur on a daily basis. It is not survival of the fittest, but survival of the most adaptive.

Fashionable fads

The world has gone mad with marketing gimmicks which use tax payer's money to support a failing system in search of a cure for many diseases. The emergence of ridiculous products with ingenious marketing strategies designed and based on false claiming miracles have arisen to persuade you into consumerism. You only have to look at weight loss products as an example. The consumer marches on like mindless sheep believing that miracles can happen in the form of a pill sold via international celebrities on prime-time television. I am baffled to hear more products produced to confuse and to win hearts of desperate people on a quest to adhere to a fashionable size. The latest gimmick; protein water and portion control plates to 'help you lose weight', apparently.

In a world where emotions are heightened, there has been significant growth addressing predominately gynaecological cancers, in an advertising practice called "pink washing". This has become so strong that many companies have jumped on this pink bandwagon, obviously for financial gain. "Pink washing", subtly advertises that a certain amount of proceeds from the purchase of goods will go to "breast cancer research". Ironically, these products contain aluminium and other nasties like parabens and certain 'numbers' that contribute significantly to formation and growth of the same cancers. Go figure!!! Walking past *'Bakers Delight'* in my own little shopping centre, I noticed a pink stand focusing on breast cancer support. The flyers clearly read "you can support Breast cancer network Australia (BCNA) by purchasing a pink finger bun between 11 May - 31 May 2017". The irony of this is that these buns are sugar, the very food that we need to avoid preventing not only cancer but obesity and diabetes! There is plenty of evidence to suggest that these sugar laden carbohydrates play a role in the development of breast cancer and other cancers. Sugar is the most acid forming food that is highly addictive with mind altering properties. Sugar leaches calcium from the bones and inhibits reabsorption, therefore, it is deposited in organs such as the kidney or on to the joints and is one of the main causes of osteoporosis. Sugar, effects the calcium-phosphorous balance, dramatically increasing triglyceride levels creating nervous hyperactivity, aggressive behaviour, cardiovascular problems, high blood pressure, digestive problems, headaches depression and anxiety. Is it any wonder that natural health practitioners refer to sugar as the "white death".

So, you can see in offering our support for this cause alone, we are supporting cancer by buying these products and unfortunately, we are brain washed and misled to falsely believe that these companies have our best health interests at heart. Although our intention is good, this action represents a huge conflict of health interest. Before you all get up in arms and start yelling out "how dare you, they are only trying to do good" .... don't shoot the messenger, because it is true!!! Shouldn't we be getting to the root of the cause in the first place? Shouldn't we be focusing on the basics of preventative methods? Should we not be supporting the person with breast cancer and the living cells of that human being? Clearing the excessive energy through oxygenating activities should be number one health priority. Plump arterial oxygenated blood can pump around your body effectively carrying nutrients to major organs like your heart and brain, from the tips of your nose to the tips of your toes. With little effort from walking clears the negative energy of lactic waste, uric acid, carbon dioxide and other poisons from our toxic lifestyles. Tissue damage and cellular health can be altered by feeding the blood correctly via clean nutrition and water making the blood less sticky and more likely to flow. It is like clearing out the old to get ready for the new.

3

FAT, FIFTY AND FINISHED?

Life is simple yet complicated! Like life, your health is the same, we over complicate it. We over think it, we overdo it and go over board to the extreme, which then makes us out of balance. In our quest to balance, we then go one step further, and out balance our attempt to balance. Self-diagnosis and self-prescribing, thanks to the internet has become more common providing imbalances and therefore creating inner turmoil.

 Give anything some form of energy and that energy will provide the growth! One negative thought can change the Course of the day….. "If you think you are beaten………. You are." For example, you have a sore on your leg. The colour changes, it starts to throb, and puss starts to ooze. It looks redder and is probably now an infection. This now may require medical intervention, probably an antibiotic. As it becomes increasingly redder, hotter (inflamed) we keep attacking it constantly picking, probing, squeezing or cutting it, yet it doesn't disappear. If we left it alone in the first place, relaxed a little and never gave it such attention it may have not become such a huge festering sore in the first place!

Our own environment, your job, friends, associates and family can keep you locked into a life that is well out of balance and beyond your control. In fact, your own inner circle can keep you 'where you are'. Because there is no manual, life is not supposed to be controlled but simply managed. To live a life bereft of any disorder, dysfunction or disease we need to realign our focus and shift our thinking from focusing on the problem to finding a solution, designed for *you.*

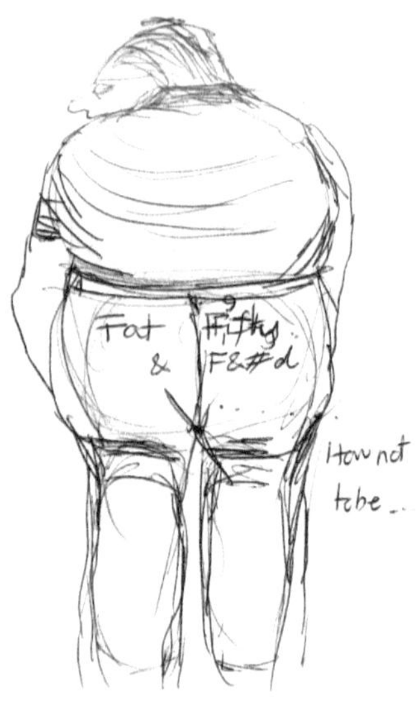

People usually move from pain to pleasure yet most people live in a whole world of pain for most of their life relying on others. Many MDs, hand out anti-depressants like lollies where really a psychologist should be seen to work through and get to the cause of their depression. From observation and in my practice, most of us are not happy or healthy, plodding monotonously through our lives like a 'steggles battery hen', meaninglessly going through the motions. Why? because it is comfortable, easy and acceptable. We crawl back into our comfort zone and drink copious of wine to drown our daily misery, or take other life altering substances to shift our thinking or we hide behind Netflix and stuff ourselves-stupid with chocolate or chips!

Who knows what's around the corner and who is to say, "it won't happen to me". Life just happens, and we react with either a crisis-management strategy or a poor- little- me- pity- party! We wander down the road without a plan and by default we end up over there when we should have been here or in another place and then wonder 'who the hell moved my cheese'?

Just imagine yourself on a beautiful ride in the mountains in the Swiss alps for a second. Your handsome husband is driving the iridescent blue BMW in the style that you are accustomed to. You are driving along nicely and quite comfortably ascending the snow-capped mountains with great speed. What seems in an instant, your cruise suddenly changes. The ascent is much greater than you had anticipated. The road becomes narrower and the weather starts closing in making visibility poor. You begin to snake through the windier roads with trepidation. The thick undergrowth of foliage that once appeared far away becomes dangerously close. The drive becomes arduous and turns from pleasurable to one of fear. A thick fog rolls in blurring your vision. As the windscreen wipers work furiously to discard the softly falling sleet, the road becomes slippery and you can feel the car sliding slightly. Taken over by fear your heart pounds wildly in your chest, your eyes widen and a thought of "shit I'm in trouble" suddenly overcomes you. Up ahead, you can barely see the road covered with impenetrable ice. To the left is a steep cliff with a jagged rock face and bare thin trees disappearing amid the fog. The attention has moved from getting there (wherever the 'there' is?) to what the f@#$ do I do now? Questions like do I slow down, take the plunge or stop the world I want to get off swim frantically round your head. The biggest question is do I Keep going the way that I am going unprepared for the consequences or am I able to take another route?

Is this the road that we want to take? Does any disease just happen like that? Should we have taken more precautionary steps before we set out on that journey? Shouldn't we have paid more attention to the signs that read "Weather may change, put on traction chains before proceeding? Should we have been more cautionary in our actions and not sped up the mountain? In any case, if and when you get to that point, "you may ask yourself what I have done and how did I get here?" Nobody just wakes up one day and suddenly announces to the world they have cancer.

If you want better health, and ultimately a better life, you may need to pay more attentions to these signs. Like the lollipop men that stand on the side of the road. They hold the signs that can alter your life. Constipation, diarrhoea, chronic flu, infections, reflux, gout, anxiety, depression, chronic pain wobbly bottoms rearing up from behind are all warning signs of danger yet to come. This may be an attempt to redirect life circumstances and make choices for better or worse. It's one thing that you are young and think, cause "that will never happen to me" but my dear friends, keep moving through the decades with a lot of these habits and trust me you will get to the point where you are not only fat but ½ a century old and unfortunately …… f&**##$d!!!

4

PREVENTION IS WAY BETTER THAN CURE.

There is no doubt that the focus on killing any disease could ultimately be our demise. Having been involved with cancer from both a theoretical and practical perspective, I have witnessed the fact that *everyone* involved, is hell bent on killing diseases that will not die yet, promote current life practices, furthering the disease continuum. There have been countless documented cases of cancer patients dying from treatment and not the cancer itself. If we change our perspective and look at all disease as one that we can live with, we may have a far greater chance of survival and outwitting any disease along with cancer.

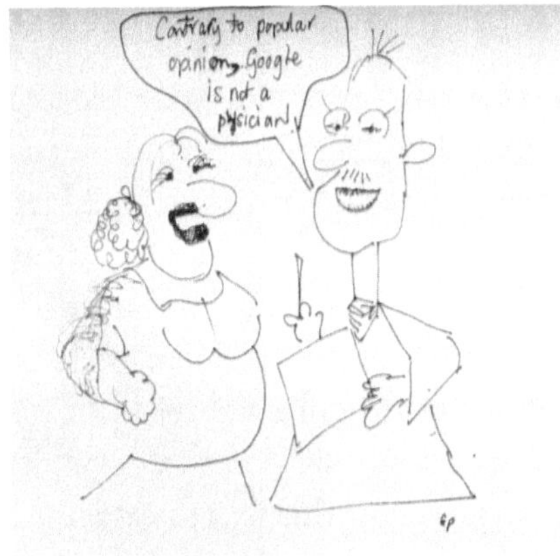

Like any drug that is prescribed, your body adapts and the dose therefore may have to be altered or increased over time to have the same efficacy. Take Lexapro, an anti-depressant for example, it will be effective for an acute period, however long-term use exacerbates symptoms to the extreme where suicidal thoughts may be entertained. To be pharmaceutical drug free by the time you reach midpoint of your life may even be an anomaly. As the body ages there is also a marked decline in the concentration, utilisation and recycling of various antioxidants such as vitamin E, C and Co-enzyme Q-10. This naturally occurring co factor production is less over 50 and has a tough time being reduced to the bioactive form (ubiquinone) which is required for energy production in all cells including heart health. The decline affects the body's ability to control free radicals, which may weaken the immune system and damage tissue such as the artery's endothelial lining. R-alpha lipoic acid, considered the master of all antioxidants helps recycle and helps extend the life of many of these vitamins and antioxidants. (4) Taking medicinal drugs that are equipped to help one disorder places enormous strain on your filtration organs so much so that they use essential vitamins and minerals needed for other chemical reactions. It is kind of like robbing Peter to give to Paul.

Other Nutrients diminish with time and from the continual perpetual stressors of life, taking the contraceptive pill and other pharmaceuticals deprive the body of essential vitamins and minerals thereby placing more stress on the body and stress, so it seems is inevitable in the world we live in. Stress, too uses the body's much needed water-soluble vitamins, B & C, leaving the body deficient. Choosing medical plants, herbs and vitamins as a substitute for a pharmaceutical may reduce the likelihood of experiencing life threatening age inducing side effects that these drugs can cause.

Although more accepting in our modern-day world, to be told you have cancer creates a sense of foreboding. For that matter mental disease is still associated with a stigma or a picture of white cladded men carrying a strait jacket assigned to restrain you. One of my cancer patients who is now 72, defied the odds of his short life sentence by adopting alternative natural medicine and an associated positive mental outlook. His rather unorthodox approach to his kidney cancer shocked his physicians as his health improved. Whilst he was afraid and anxious he could not allow this fear to get on top of him. He said once you gave way to fear, you are gone! Many people fall into a state of depression from this fear. This fear of the unknown may lead to a decreased immune system driving a diseased state. Fear, depression or aggression! Aggression leads to War and the concept of fighting a war within our own bodies is beyond logical. To whom are we fighting? Are we fighting to defend life, against the enemy? But who and what is the enemy? The ultimate enemy is death. Yet, all men must die ...... <u>V</u>alar Morghulis!

"Darkness cannot drive out darkness, only light can do that. Hate cannot drive out hate, only love can do that."

Martin Luther King.

The "war" on cancer was initiated in 1971 by President Nixon. Embarking on an advertising campaign with the slogan "Mr Nixon, you can cure cancer". An additional 100 mill USD for cancer research was employed. Whilst billions of dollars have been poured into "killing this disease", we are no closer to finding any solution than we were sixty years ago. The paper headlines read ... New hope ...... new cure ... new drug. Commercial television provides us with insightful revelations of such miracle drugs yet predominately cancer patients arrive in their thousands turning up to an unchanged fate and it isn't pretty! Only just the other day I sat with a 67-year-old patient in his own home. His brown weathered stick insect appearance bore the results of chemotherapy, yet he defied that his treatment was not killing him. Being of European descent, living on stodgy food, living with toxic chemicals all of his working life, a heavy smoker and a chronic alcoholic, it did not come as a surprise that liver cancer was his primary! His prognosis was grim and now metastatic. He was still convinced that his oncologist was going to give him another chance at life. He was on heavy pain medication due to an infection that had arisen after his whipple surgery. He could hardly swallow and when he could, due to the nausea caused by the pain killers on an empty stomach, he threw them all up! A catch 22, double edged sword scenario. The call to a nutritionist at this point is almost futile, however to feed him spoons of wholesome goodness to assist his body to heal is the only thing that one can do. In such cases, it is all too late, the horse has already bolted! It was too late. He died about a fortnight after.

The war waged on disease and the ultimate disease, cancer, quote, "...Is the biggest international lie that has been fed to our society". These words are not my own but from one of my patient's carers. I am only the conduit between the real people that are fed up with being fed with incorrect material. So, if we are at war, when did the war begin, who are we fighting and what are we fighting for? One of the greatest legendary military strategist Sun Tzu, author of the most infamous book "The art of war" believed in fighting battles where the odds were in his favour. He explains that "an army's opportunities come from openings in the environment caused by the relative weakness of the enemy". (5) Here lies the difference between what natural practitioners and traditional medical intervention does. *Natural herbs and medical foods assist the bodies healing process, traditional medicine aims to stop by killing not only the disorder, but the very person itself.*

For arguments sake, If we are to fight a war on disease, then let's consider the cell being the army and the diseased tissue, the enemy. Shouldn't we be focusing on developing the strength of our army by building an impregnable environment that provides resistance to our enemy. If we respected our bodies, ate generally clean-living foods, walked far from cars and close to nature, lived a stress-free life or stressed less, we would be nourishing our army and toxic to the enemy. James Duke, herbal botanist with a string of heathy plant promoting books including the green pharmacy made an interesting comment in his book 'Anti-aging prescriptions', he said "to maintain a disease-free state we have to become flexible in all areas of our life". This is our life and a glimpse of the disease continuum, the fact that we are constantly changing, we may as well be prepared for the changes that will happen anyway. (6)

The cancer war concept is ongoing focusing on killing something that lives within us overlooking that all diseases, including cancer is within us and is actually a part of the sum total of us. Conflict, confusion poisons and potions raging in and outside our body, what chance has our personal army got to defend itself against any enemy? Nipping any disorder in the bud is so much easier than the latter. Believe me, it is in our best interest to say the least to avoid the peril of any disease like cancer that has no cure, regardless of what you hear, listen to or read! It all begins with us and at any age we can intervene!

Having said that we can learn to live our lives with love, joy, adopting old age natural remedies and philosophies that have stood the testament of time. Coming from a love-based perspective, not a fear based one, we then too will have a renewed respect for this precious body that we all have been given. It is not as easy task, given the society in which we live but when has there ever been a perfect society?

> "He who is well prepared and lies in wait for an enemy who is not well prepared will win"
>
> Sun Tzu, the art of War.

Rule 101 in practising medicine in any form is to stay emotionally detached. Even still being in the trenches alongside metastatic patients can and often break your heart. After determining the special nutrient needs of a middle-aged woman with metastatic brain cancer, I became entrenched in her life. Learning of her tragic story expressed my sympathy and stepped beyond the boundaries of practice as I cooked and delivered food for herself and her family. Her needs exceeded my own. There was no one else that could help, and I wanted to see her eat. I really believed it was not necessarily food that she needed. It was, in fact, the one crucial ingredient missing from her life, and that was love. Buddha said that there are primarily only two things in life that people need, and that is to be productive and to be loved. This woman heralded the loudest tune sung in our society today .... **loneliness**! She was merely a carcass of a woman, barely skin and bone! I quickly discovered that she more than likely, was an alcoholic, as her preference for champagne, over rode her choice to eat and provided an escape from her reality!

Her life was miserable. Her daughter was in jail which left her two grandchildren in her sole care. Her emaciated body was literally being eaten alive and every day I could see changes in her failing mind. Originally diagnosed with Small cell lung cancer(SCLC), at the advice of her oncologist many years before, had taken the normal route of therapy. It was expensive chemo initially, and with this option failing she then relied on integrated doctors for intravenous vitamin C. She had done everything that she could think of within her means to cure herself, except eat real food and change her *very* stressful life. I often think this odd, how can anyone endure any disease let alone vile treatment without the help of basic energy requirements. I was her last port of call, her final desperate attempt at clutching to the threads of life. But, once again it was too late. The communication between us became less as her speech and thought processes failed. Within a few months, after several unsuccessful attempts to contact her, she had found her peaceful resting place. Caring for two active grandchildren aged 5 and 6 in a small and humble 2-bedroom apartment on a meagre pension took its toll. Drinking pure sugar every night to numb her existence and even admitting that she would rather die than be denied that pleasure, was her icing on her cake! I guess it was her choices that determined her outcome!

It was this experience that had a profound effect on me and it was then I decided that I wanted to work with patients that said yes to life. It also changed the direction of how I wanted to practice nutritional and holistic medicine. It also reinforced the fact that "prevention is far easier than cure."

It's hard to imagine that giving a few herbs, providing nutrient dense foods and to get moving is that we who practice natural medicine, can be such a threat to powerful global prosperous pharma companies. Still, people are fed up with being sick and not getting the answers from these powerful authorities. In fact, they are sick and tired of being sick and more people are looking to the past in search of a simpler more authentic and more importantly a healthier way to live their lives. It seems that health and medicine has become invariably divided and the words health and care has been eliminated from our health care. Desmond Dos said it all whilst performing his acts of love in a chaotic bloody war "whilst everyone *is taking life I am going to save some*". That's the aim, to restore order within chaos … and it can be done. *It may involve a bit of tweaking.* Better to live and die by your own sword, rather than somebody else's!

Whilst the analogy of war is a tad overdone, this is not war and therefore we should not reduce ourselves to be fighting, someone or something, a disorder or a disease that already exists within. We are not a standalone entity. We are human beings consisting of a symbiotic relationship between the mind, body and spirit and therefore we exist in this physical world as such. To treat chronic disease like mental health autoimmune and cancer cannot be separated from those three criteria. Emotionally, intelligently intertwined the body deserves to be treated with the utmost respect like a first-time lover delicately fingering the contours of the body. It is the imbalances between these criteria that affect our bodies and our lives which ultimately leads to growth of a destructive emotional or physical beast.

Life emits energy and the amount of energy given to kill disease, especially cancer is extravagant and time consuming to the point of obsessive. My interactions with many metastatic patients left me thinking why they would want to put themselves through this and why did they want to live at all. They blamed the Doctor that did not "pick it up as early as it should have", or the fact that they were not given the right treatment. No one ever mentioned that they themselves may have been responsible for their outcome. Many of them expressed anger and resentment and an apparent lack of love for others and themselves. At that point, it got me thinking. Is a lack of self-love one of the drivers of disease? Or is it that we do not care or are we not prepared?

The five Ps of life

"It isn't what we say or think that defines us but what we do ……"

Jane Austen.

After failing time after time in various instances in my life, lessons have been learnt the hard way. As being guilty as charged unless you perfect the lesson, life will continually deal the same lesson until you get it!! Get it???? After speaking in public at a National conference only last year on the effects of nutrients on Gut health, I am afraid to say, "I choked". After telling one of my sisters, who is a public speaker and teacher at the academy of Police in Queensland, of my horrific failure, she sniggered and told me I had forgotten the 5 "Ps"; I looked at her blankly, I had no idea as to what she was speaking about when she blurted out; "poor preparation promotes pitiful performance". Some say, piss-weak preparation promotes piss-poor performance. Whichever way you look at it, it is still failing! Without taking the time to prepare and plan properly, you can fail. In fact, without using these 5 Ps can set you up to fail not only in a presentation, business, but strangely enough our health and our life! Nobody, in their right mind, builds a house without a sturdy foundation. Marriage too, needs a solid foundation based on certain criteria. Love, trust and respect amongst others. These ingredients are fundamentals just like your health, holding you in good stead to weather unexpected storms!

It is not new that we have reached health proportions of a crisis point. Escalating obesity, high blood pressure, asthma, chronic pain, depression, anxiety, constipation, hormonal havoc and desensitised immune systems. There seems to be a sense of hopelessness beguiling our modern-day life even as young as teenage years. Australia and most of the western world perceived to be the more developed nations spend more on 'health care' yet still has the worst state of both physical and mental health. Whilst Primitive nations that exist primarily on a subsistence level are free of these western diseases that seem to be strangling our children, youth and adults.

Anxiety and depression are stepping out in the limelight and becoming the new diseases of this century and one of our biggest problems is constipation. Who would have thought something so natural would become so hard? (pun unintended) It is not ok to poop only once a week which is the advice offered from midwives, to young mothers after sharing concerns about their children's bowel habits. Constipation may even refer to a person that poops daily, let alone a whole week! I do not understand how this can be ok and if this is what we are teaching our young, god help the future! Your poop tells more than you think about your health and if you strain, grunt and groan or worse, have trouble getting to the throne, then there may be something a little off or damaged, leading to other profound consequences later. Remember the digestive tract is just a passage. The only open-ended system in our body, a tube that starts at the mouth and ends up in the southern orifice, your anus. Hard to imagine that a simple act can alleviate many problematic symptoms of ill health so let it go and let it flow. It really is that simple … Great health is basic. Eat, sleep, move and poop!

Speaking of hard so many of our young men suffering from penile erectile dysfunction is more common than you think. If you can hit

40 and have that old boy stand up to attention without any assistance from a pill, consider yourself lucky! The mount of droopers and less sexually active engaged couples is alarming to say the least. Something so natural and pleasurable has become an arduous task. Men can't, and women can't be bothered!

5

IS OUR MODERN-DAY DIET KILLING US?

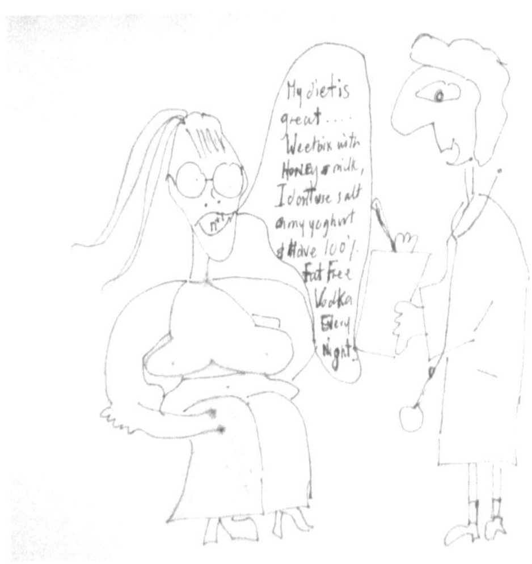

*"When diet is wrong medicine is of no use. When
diet is correct medicine is of no need ".*

There is nothing refined about refined food and refined food is, definitely, not refined! International health took a dramatic decline when refined and processed foods were introduced. The rise of degenerative disease and diabetes correlates with the rise in consumption of foods that have all the nutrients stripped out with harmful preservatives and additives packaged in. Modern agriculture and processing techniques have not advanced our health at all with an overabundance of processed combination of monosaccharide, disaccharides, polysaccharides, trans fat, additives and preservatives. Sugar is sugar and can be hidden, wrapped in attractive plastic packages. Disguised by strange chemical names combined with unusual compounds of preservatives and unidentifiable additives that require a dictionary to decipher. Sucrolose, an artificial sweetener found in splenda may cause shrunken thymus glands, skin rashes and enlarged liver and kidneys. Tartrazine, a food colouring, may be petroleum derived, causing urticaria, asthma, allergic reactions, hypertension and anaphylaxis. The Diabetes Association of Australia advocates that it is ok, ironically to use sucrolose and acesulfame potassium (950) used in soft drinks, jelly, dips, snacks, sauces and toppings. These have been reported to produce tumours, leukaemia and chronic respiratory disease in animal related studies. (7) This baffles me as whilst these so called nutritional experts condone these unnecessary items, they also say to stay away from <u>fruit due to its high fructose content</u>. Fruit in its natural state provides more nutrients in the way of phytochemicals and phyto-nutrients that the body recognises and can utilise, just the way nature intended. No wonder many people are confused.

Foods containing trans fats, sugars, chemicals that cannot be pronounced with so many numbers, leads to a disproportionate di-obesity, fat and sick problem on an international platform. Processed food whilst attractive and appealing promotes universal health problems in the form of undesirable disorders ranging from issues with digestion, metabolic disease, obesity and cancer. These carcinogenic toxins have snuck into our diets through aggressive marketing tactics. Progress? Advancement? I am not totally convinced!

It is truth that in today's modern world we have replaced the concept of fresh and organic with fast and convenient. If we are totally honest about our food choices, we may be abusing that liberty. Convenience and taste may be our killers. Most of us lack the time, so we do whatever we do to relieve hunger or to satisfy our taste buds. If that means cheese and bikkies with a glass of wine when we get home from a hard day in the office, we do. Grabbing a ham & cheese croissant while we fill up at the local BP, on the way to and from work, we do. We do what we do because it works. But sooner or later, (hopefully later than sooner) this type of eating will catch up with us and probably not in a good way. Food is fuel, but is this the fuel that we need? To promote vitality and health in all aspects in our lives we need to have the necessary ingredients. Today our food choices "just ain't cutting it!" Gorging on foods sitting for hours in a bay-Marie & sipping calorically dense caramel lattes mid-morning is doing us more harm than good. Sitting in front of electromagnetic devices day in and day out squashing vital organs is slowly killing us.

We do not have to wander far to see that obesity and diabetes is an epidemic. You are more likely to find a herd of friendly hippopotami at a table, devouring mountainous plates of unnecessary and unidentified calories at the local food court than on a David Attenborough's African plain's story. If you think that's harsh, then go to Bali and see the epidemic of fat in a third world country. I felt sorry for the poor bikes that carry hefty bottoms through the foul polluted and un-eco-friendly suburbs of Kuta, Legian and Seminyak. In women's clothing, the new 8 is now a size 12, and god forbid we let anyone in on that secret! Excess weight may be an issue initially, but it is the extra burden on highly important organs like the pancreas, liver, gall bladder and heart that is impacted over time. It then becomes all too hard to get off the arm chair to even change the channel and these days, we thank god for the remote as who need legs any way, they are so yesterday!! Not!!

Feeding your body fatty foods laden with sugar gives the body energy but that energy if not used and deleted gets stored as fat. We are all guilty, practitioners included. We keep on stuffing the body with a plethora of "stuff" and the result is that you either become stuffed or you "get stuffed". We need to move more and eat less, it really is that simple!!!

> "If medicine wants to focus on prevention there is no better tool than nutrition".

Dominic d'Agostino

Food has been used as medicine for thousands of years in the treatment of so many disorders with a great deal of success, yet when it comes to treatment to any disorder, it is far easier to take a pill than changing a bad habit. If we look closely at any dysfunction and the continuum of disease progression they all have to come from something. A bacterium, a bug, a virus, the environment, the foods we eat or the foods that we don't eat. Our current dietary practices, our modern-day lifestyle and the lack of physical exercise are probably, by far the most common cause of awakening the monster within.

6

DIGESTION BEGINS
IN THE KITCHEN

If we have to start somewhere in restoring health, then let's look at the process of digestion. The kitchen is still, probably one of the busiest places in the household. A central meeting point, a drawing card for the famished and contrary to popular opinion, the starting point of digestion. I find myself drawn to conversations engaging in the joy of cooking for those that you love. One of the long-lost bastions of a tradition we have known as home cooking has been usurped by the conveniences of frequent take outs and dining out as an alternative. A sign of the times yet this one simple change in our lifestyle may have profound effects on our health, our digestion.

Once upon a time, when my own children were small, the children fought over homemade cakes that I would prepare for them in the afternoon and then squabble over stools, positioning themselves at the bench whilst I cut, sliced, diced and threw concoctions of food together to feed the masses! No matter what I cooked, even if it was sausages and vegetables they still asked me what the hell it was! However just like a good red wine, my culinary skills and nutritional knowledge has expanded somewhat, and I am proud to say, my cooking is deliciously palatable, balanced and full of high density nutrition.

Somewhere between then and now, we have lost the art of the cooking process. From the selection of the meats, to the choices of vegetables, herbs and spices that enhance the flavour. Cooking at home is more than just about filling up on food as fuel, with benefits, unfortunately omitted. Once we open the fridge, begin to choose the produce and slowly start the simmer broiling or baking process the waft of culinary delights, incite our sensory perception, stimulating our taste buds, kick starting digestion.

For busy mums, their role as a taxi service seems to weave in and around that time when normally a family would sit down at a dining table and have their evening meal together. It is not uncommon that this important meal is skipped. If we ask most families where they eat their meals, I am 100% sure their response would be, watching television or in front of their computer. Digestion starts before we even sit down, let alone once we start the process of mastication.

It all starts with the smell and taste, then the mechanism of digestion begins. When we put food into our mouths, natures plan is that we are supposed to chew thoroughly to liquid, a process called mastication. Chewing is not simply to make swallowing easier. As we chew, saliva lubricates the food and amylase, a digestive enzyme is released in the mouth to assist the breakdown of carbohydrates. Without this action, our bodies would not be able to assimilate the valuable vitamins and minerals that are necessary for our bodies to run. The less time chewing may result in straining the next part of digestion. Poor chewing can mean less amylase. Once the food reaches the stomach other enzymes are released by the pancreas. These are responsible for dissembling the proteins and fats which are further broken down and absorbed in the intestines. Gulping down glasses of water in-between each bite may confuse the body further and increase burping and discomfort after eating. Water may also decrease the much-needed hydrochloric acid required to catabolise these macronutrients. A rushed meal with no preparation from being time poor, could result in digestive discomfort with bloating, burping, farting and starting with undigested food particles showing up in your stools. If digestion does not go according to plan, then even at this early stage it's probably likely that you won't be able to fully digest the meal and take the available nourishment from it. Ironically, take out may be a poor time management decision after all.

One of the worst foods that have been created and packaged and then consumed by our infants are the squishy mass produced and highly processed fruit and vegetable liquids sold in our supermarkets. Whilst young mothers consciously consider that this is a better snack option, than chips, cakes and biscuits, these choices are creating other problems such as poor teeth development. Some children are not learning to chew and are missing out on the benefits of this simple exercise. This could even set them up for gastrointestinal disturbances and a compromised immune system. Food should be fresh, seasonal and alive with raw enzymes fuelling sustainable nutrients for their immune function, growth and brain formation.

Whilst we are on the subject of 'alive', the greatest innovation within a kitchen, the microwave is one of the deadliest devices used in households today. Microwaves are a form of electromagnetic radiation posing harmful health implications although some scientific websites and articles refute this entirely. Radiation within this device causes destruction and changes of molecules within food. Here lies the problem, the result is the formation of radiolytic compounds which are unknown to man and nature.

The solution to this story is simple. Get engaged in the kitchen. More time spent in the kitchen preparing and planning our meals surrounded by loved ones can mean a more efficient digestive system. It is an activity that brings joy and one to be treasured. If only we could get back to basics, it may protect the generation to come, that is if we honour our future and the future of our children's.

7

YOUR GUT- THE HIGHWAY OF LIFE!

According to the Collins Dictionary , "Instinct, is the natural tendency that a person or animal has to behave or react in a particular way". (11) The phrase "trust your gut", is your body, alerting you to something that is either ok or not quite right. If it does not sit right, your body will tell you via pain, or a sickening feeling like the impact from a kick in the guts. Oh, oh, body this is a Code 3 alert! If that's the case, then you are probably right. If we all trusted our natural instincts, we would be a whole lot better off. One of the forefathers of medicine, Hippocrates once said "All disease starts in the gut" so I guess that fixing this issue may be the best place to start.

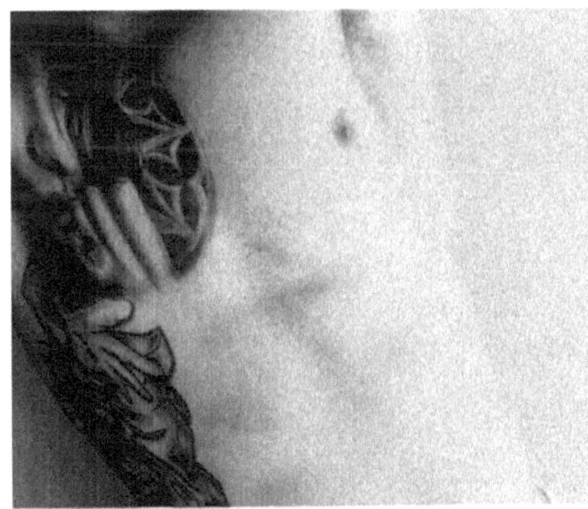

It is hard to believe that with all the valuable information floating on the "cloud", that the world is still in a state of confusion. Never, before, have we seen so many people that have a distressed and disordered digestive system. There has been substantial evidence that reveals immune dysfunction, obesity, rheumatoid arthritis, autism, depression, chronic fatigue syndrome, mental illness, diabetes and cancer can be alleviated by improving our gut health. The gut is the second brain. The gut brain axis is a definitive link between the gut and the brain which is basically a super highway that links the gut, gut flora, nervous system and the hypothalamic-pituitary-adrenal axis. It is a two-way biochemical communication system occurring via the vagus nerve and the mechanisms including the neuro - immune - endocrine mediators. This explains how our thoughts and feelings and stress can impact our gut sensations, motility and secretions. All, of our sensations arising in the gut can impact the brain, leading to changes in our mood, behaviour, cognitive function, motivation and pain.

For arguments sake, that "gut feeling", could be associated with a condition called "leaky gut". A recurring and growing epidemic often presenting in loads of people but misdiagnosed as another disorder or disease. Leaky gut has many associations with various symptoms like bloating, candida overgrowth, constipation or ongoing diarrhoea even nasty bouts of flatulence.

But what is it and why are so many people plagued from these symptoms? Leaky gut is intestinal permeability or hyper-permeability, a consequence of *intestinal tight junction* malfunction. Intestinal junctions in the lining of your intestines are normally knitted together to form a kind of mesh that acts as a protective barrier between the digestive tract and your fluids. Food, gut microbiota, toxins, incomplete undigested proteins and fats leak through these broken junctions or gaps into the surrounding fluid and tissue causing inflammation. Ironically enough inflammation causes this mesh to break and allow this to occur in the first place. If the gut cannot properly digest nutrients and these particles escape this may be the root cause of other disorders. A leaking gut may occur at any point but is definitely from what you put or don't put into your mouth.

Symptoms may spread body wide causing systemic inflammation which could be attributed to other lifestyle factors such as stress. Stress then affects digestion which then furthers more inflammation. The gaps widen due to inflammation which leads to further malabsorption and a myriad of other disorders like headaches, migraines, joint pain, thyroid issues, weight gain, fatigue, depression and immune dysfunction. When inflammation is present, your immune system normally comes to the rescue sending out a team of killer cells that attack the pathogens that are not recognised as friendly to the system. The challenge is by doing this they inadvertently attack healthy cells in the process furthering more inflammation. It is a tangled web we weave.

One of the two related variables determining our gut health or "gut flora" is the microbiota and the gut barrier. Our gut is home to approximately <u>100 trillion microorganisms</u>. The human gut contains 10 times more bacteria than all the human cells in the entire body, with over 400 known diverse bacterial specie. The gut flora promotes normal gastrointestinal function, provides protection from infection, regulates metabolism and comprises more than 75% of our immune system. Dysregulated gut flora has been linked to diseases ranging from autism and depression to autoimmune conditions like Hashimoto's, inflammatory bowel disease and type 1 diabetes. Unfortunately, our modern-day diet and life style can promote dysregulation in our microbiota. Constant antibiotic use, (by the way means anti-life), various medications and birth control pills contribute to this imbalance. Chronic stress, diets high in processed foods, diets low in fermentable fibres, dietary toxins like wheat and industrial seed oils may contribute to a leaky gut, irritable bowel disorders such as crohns, and ulcerative colitis. According to Functional Medical practitioner Chris Kresser, M.S., L.Ac, there are primarily four common food toxins that are largely responsible for the epidemic of modern diseases that are destroying our health. These four toxins are Wheat, sugar, industrial seed oil, and surprise, surprise, Soy! (12) Speaking of oils, I am often confused at what is deemed a health snack? A quest bar, a protein bar that is sold in commercial supermarkets and health food stores clearly label the contents which adds Palm oil. Apart from having environmental issues, this oil is a saturated fat contributing to weight gain. It is a misconception that because it is in the health isle of our supermarket that this product is considered "healthy".

The overuse of antibiotics has been known to shift the diversity and composition of the natural gut flora meaning that we need to intervene to pop back the gut flora. An old concept of weeding and feeding has been used in the naturopathic world when we speak of gut health as we compare our gut to a garden which needs constant care.

It has been repeatedly shown in several well-designed studies that the integrity of the intestinal barrier is a major factor in autoimmune disease. Leaky gut and bad gut flora are common because of the modern lifestyle. If you have a leaky gut, you probably have bad gut flora and if you have bad gut flora then you probably too have a leaky gut! When your gut flora and gut barrier are impaired, you will be inflamed. Inflammation leads to disease, period. Since gut health is now recognised by general Medical Doctors as being a major contributor to modern day diseases a critical molecule called zonulin is a culprit. Zonulin opens the spaces between the cells of the intestinal lining. This normally occurs, in order for nutrient and other molecules to get in and out of the intestine. When the levels of zonulin increase, the seal between the intestinal cells close giving room between the cell that allow everything to pass right through. Sometimes large food molecules will pass through to the immune system. The immune system thinks they are foreign invaders and will mount an immune response leading to food sensitivities. In addition, this immune activation leads to more damage to the intestinal cells (called enterocytes) and the gut becomes more inflamed and more permeable or "leaky". As the damage continues, the microvilli that line the intestines and absorb nutrients become damaged, leading to other nutrient deficiencies. (13)

Two most powerful triggers to open the zonulin door are *gluten and gut bacteria* in the small intestine. A few causes of increased zonulin and a development of a leaky gut may be due to an overgrowth of harmful organisms like bacteria and yeast in the intestine, SIBO (small intestinal bacterial overgrowth), fungal dysbiosis or candida overgrowth and parasite infections. Auto immune disease, including celiac, multiple sclerosis, type 1 diabetes, rheumatoid arthritis and hashimotos are characterised by abnormally high levels of zonulin with a leaky gut being responsible. (14)

The good news is that we can fix the problem with a little work from you and mend the gaps, get you back to absorbing the nutrients from your food so that you will feel better and subsequently live a rather normal unaffected life. Here is a five-part protocol to resurrect your GIT and to allow the flow of food to create the energy for you to feel well again. Let's review an ancient protocol to treat any inflammatory bowel condition. Alternative health practitioners have a version of this in addition to what is on offer. Here is a 5-step practice that may play an enormous role in healing your gut issues so that farting and starting does not play out in your day!

The five-part protocol to gut health;

Eliminate; Establish, experiment, equalise & evacuate,

1. Eliminate

If something is causing you pain the most obvious thing to do is to get rid of it. So eliminate any short chain carbohydrates like lactose found in milk and fructose contained in fruit. Furthermore, work towards avoiding foods that contain **Fructans,** found in gluten grains like wheat, spelt, rye and barley. Fructans can be also found in dried fruits such as dates, pineapple & raisins. Stay away from **Galactan** compounds found in substantial amounts in legumes. Get rid of the **Polyols:** These are the sugar alcohols like xylitol, sorbitol, maltitol and mannitol. We need to avoid these as they most probably are responsible for bouts of distension, flatulence, and an unfortunate odour! Mind you this could be due to poor absorption. Or worse, a subsequent osmotic effect meaning that they draw liquid into the intestine, causing unwanted diarrhoea. When the undigested saccharide reaches the colonic flora, it is quickly metabolised to produce hydrogen and carbon dioxide and produced too quickly for the body to metabolise or pass, abdominal distension and pain are often the result. (15)

Avoid, proteins found in unsprouted grains, sugar, genetically modified organisms or GMOs and conventional dairy. These common components of food can damage your intestinal lining. These proteins contain nutrient blockers called lectins and phytates. Both phytates and lectins are plant toxins binding to vitamins and minerals in turn making those nutrients bio-unavailable. Sugar binding protein such as lectin attach to the digestive lining causing damage to your GIT, irritation and inflammation!

Conventional cow's milk is another food that may cause leaky gut due to the pasteurization process and the protein, A1 casein. Pasteurising destroys vital enzymes including lactase, making it difficult for lactose to be digested properly. Alternatively, raw milk, A2 cow's milk, goat, sheep, camel and buffalo could be used instead. Lactose is the sugar of milk and too much impairs the body's ability to metabolise sugar.

Good old sugar is yet another substance that seems to always rear its ugly head in disturbing the natural order of digestion. Sugar in many forms feed the growth of yeast, candida and bad and unwanted bacteria furthering the damage to your gut. Exotoxins are synthesized by the bad bacteria which chomp on the lining of the GIT, creating gaps furthering the damage of the intestines.

Stress is also a major player exacerbating symptoms of all these diseases, whilst mostly self-manifested a better option is to learn to manage it before it seriously manages you. Get rid of the nagging wife or husband, kids or job or whatever it is that is causing you stress in the first place (only kidding !!) better still just learn to calm down and learn to think differently to cope with the current situation. Ask yourself every day before that trigger is pulled on that loaded gun of classic explosive histrionics, "is this life threatening, and will it matter tomorrow?"

2 **establish with** healing foods

Bone broth My first go to for people suffering from any of the above presenting complaints is good old fashioned clear fluid with animal bones. Bone broth is not only delicious but contains collagen and specific amino acids like proline and glycine helping to heal the intestinal lining. A must for auto- immune disease. If you are serious about healing have a 3 day fast of bone broth alone then introduce other foods back into your diet. Food that have nutritious healing properties like vegetables steamed with a small parcel of protein. Small quantities at first and note the action or rather the reaction!

Raw Cultured Dairy Small chain fatty acids (SCFA's) are an important source of energy for cells in the GIT. SCFAS produce butyrate acid, a fatty acid important for gut-related diseases from autoimmunity to obesity to colon cancer. Butyrate helps control the growth of the cells lining the gut, to make sure there's good balance between old cells dying and new cells being formed. Specialised dairy products like kefir, butter, goat's yoghurt and raw cheese that contain probiotics and small chain fatty acids (SCFA's) help to heal the gastro intestinal pipeline.

SCFA Food Sources

The following soluble dietary fibre produces most SCFA in the large intestine

- <u>Resistant starches</u> from whole-grain cereals, barley, brown rice, beans, lentils, green bananas, cooked and cooled potatoes or pasta
- <u>Pectin</u> from apples, apricots, blackberries, carrots and oranges
- <u>Fructo oligosaccharides (FOS)</u> and <u>inulin</u> from Jerusalem artichokes, leeks, rye and asparagus.

Fermented Vegetables – contain organic acids that balance intestinal pH and probiotics to support the gut. Sauerkraut, kimchi are excellent sources, growing in popularity and more readily available in all major health food stores today.

Coconut Products – Generally speaking most **coconut** products are especially good for your gut. The Medium chain fatty acids (MCFA's) in coconut are easier to digest than other fats so they work well for a leaking gut. Also, coconut kefir contains probiotics that support your digestive system.

Sprouted Seeds – chia seeds, flaxseeds and hemp seeds that have been sprouted are great sources of fibre that can help support the growth of beneficial bacteria. If you have severe leaky gut, you may need to start out getting your fibre from steamed vegetables and some fruit.

Omega 3 fats. Fat is your friend and sugar is the enemy is consistent amongst functional medical Doctors. Consuming foods that have omega-3 fats are beneficial to the GIT as they contain anti-inflammatory properties. Beneficial amino acids contained in grass-fed beef, lamb and wild-caught fish like salmon.

Experiment with specific supplements

Digestive enzymes

An easy solution to the disordered digestive system and constipation may be as easy as taking a supplemental digestive enzyme. Unless you eat raw foods at the beginning of every meal like pineapple pieces that contain bromelain or papaya containing the natural enzyme papain that will assist catabolic reactions, these enzymes will be highly beneficial when taken in supplementary form for a cyclic period of course! Digestive enzymes at the beginning of each meal ensure all foods are completely digested. If your stools indicate fragments of food, it is highly likely that you need these. By taking digest-ymes it decreases the chance that partially digested food particles and proteins will damage your gut wall.

L-Glutamine

Supplementation has been critical for any program designed to heal leaky gut and to improve the GUT integrity. **Glutamine powder** is an essential amino acid supplement that is anti-inflammatory and necessary for the growth and repair of your intestinal lining. L-glutamine benefits include acting as a protector: coating your cell walls and acting as a repellent to irritants. Take 2–5 grams twice daily.

Slippery elm

Native to the North Americans The Red Elm is best known for its gelatinous bark powder, slippery elm. It has been used as a herbal remedy for hundreds of years restoring gut health in general. The healing mucilage properties inflates in the digestive system to provide a protective barrier soothing irritation while absorbing toxins. It also has anti-inflammatory effects protecting the integrity of the membrane lining.

Apple pectin.

Whilst the go to is preferably an organic apple the pectin found in apples has been effective to relieve digestive complaints associated with leaky gut and irritable bowel conditions.

Quercetin

One of my favourite nutrients shown to improve gut barrier function. By assisting the creation of tight junction proteins, it seals the gut. It also stabilizes mast cells and reduces the release of histamine, common in food intolerance. Histamine overload cause allergic-type reactions like sneezing, wheezing, asthma, runny noses, watery eyes and skin rashes. It acts like a natural histamine, when taken with other nutrients like vitamin C, Rutin and bioflavonoids. Novel studies have also shown its effectiveness in healing ulcerative colitis. Take 500 milligrams three times daily with meals.

Aloe Vera

Traditionally known for its use on skin complaints it is brilliantly helpful for the relief of skin aggravations caused by excessive histamine activation internally. It aids absorption of the vitamins and minerals within your diet and any supplements you may be taking.

Turmeric

Turmeric has made a huge comeback over the last two to three years for relief of pro inflammatory disorders. Turmeric contains Bioactive Compounds called curcuminoids with powerful Medicinal Properties. It is a Natural Anti-Inflammatory Compound and dramatically increases the antioxidant capacity of the body. It has been called an anti-aging nutrient for this very reason. Having only a half-life of about 15 minutes, research has shown that combined with a phospholipid (fat) it by passes the watery intestines, staying longer in the body with improved efficacy. Combined with other herbs like boswellia and salix alba or white willow bark, they all work in unison to down regulate inflammation, reduce fever and pain. It is commonly used in the treatment of many disorders including arthritis, back pain and fibromyalgia. In the past years it has also been utilised in the treatment of some cancers intravenously.

Implement and experiment with the help of a natural practitioner to provide the combination, the dosage and the frequency of use.

Equalise

If we imagine our gut like a garden, we then understand that like every garden it needs to be tended with love and care. Spraying the garden with weed killer will kill those pesky weeds that grow with gay abandon whilst the flowers become strangled by their strong and ever-growing presence. Spraying weed killer is like giving your gut an anti-biotic, sure it will kill off the weeds or the bad bacteria, but it will also kill any good and protective bacteria.

A probiotic is 'prolife, in other words Taking a probiotic promotes life. A probiotic with specific strains can be one of the most important supplements replenishing beneficial bacteria while crowding out bad bacteria, therefore an equaliser. Probiotic foods too contain live bacteria, which may help restore balance and offer protection from harmful bacteria. Eating them is one way to reseed your gut with healthy bacteria as your diet sustains your gut bacteria. A study performed on mice indicated that oral administration of the strain Lactobacillus acidophilus (L.A) can alter the cytokine production in tumour bearing mice reducing tumour growth and increasing lymphocyte proliferation. This translates to having a favourable anti-tumour effect especially in breast cancer. (16) More and more studies have emerged with new and encouraging evidence in support of the use of probiotics to redesign our microbiota. Probiotics has the ability to prevent and reduce the incidence of common illnesses including neurodegenerative disease such as Parkinson's. To make your life a little easier, choose a probiotic that restores digestive function after use of antibiotics. Science is forever changing and 2016 saw a pronounced growth in the development of probiotics and with a huge compilation of evidence to suggest that a multi-spectrum of various species strengthens the immune system, promotes healthy bowel movements, relieves, constipation, improves IBS, symptoms, reduces the symptoms of eczema, prevents yeast infections, improves nutrient absorption, reduces, inflammation and gut permeability and generally supports optimal health and well-being! I guess that is what we are aiming for!

Microbiome and the effect on weight.

Any one that has ever had an interest in losing weight and not been successful after so many attempts at being on the roller coaster ride of yo-yo dieting may be interested in this. Higher amount of certain types of gut microbes within the gut may contribute to your ability to either increase weight significantly or decrease your ability to lose weight. Researchers through numerous studies found that those that spent time yo-yo dieting decreased their gut microbiome diversity, which led them to believe that altered microbes were probably the reason of weight gain. Lean people on the other hand, have a more diverse range of microbe specimen. A nine-year study that involve 1532 female twins exemplified this fact, since they were twins, the weight gain or loss could be how weight gain does not have to do with genetic factors. Only 4 % of change in weight could be attributed to genes meaning that other factors in addition to a higher intake of calories and genetics play in the role of obesity, being overweight or being lean. Sleep deprivation is another causative factor in obesity and weight gain not considered here and a completely different story. Microbiome targeting approaches to reduce metabolic aberrations assist in promoting weight stability. (17)

So what comes first the probiotic or the prebiotic. In short prebiotics are the non-digestible carbohydrates that act as fuel for probiotics. A prebiotic is normally a specialized plant fibre like inulin a constituent in globe artichoke that beneficially nourishes the beneficial bacteria already in the large bowel or colon. Use foods in its raw forms with easily digestible proteins with healthy fats, then use a probiotic with about 35 billion CFUs. Since, last year alone more superior quality probiotics are in the market place with multi strains and up to 500 billion CFUs. Choose a multigenerational broad-spectrum probiotic that has a combination of scientifically proven strains. This means that they work synergistically to proliferate a dynamic flora within the gastrointestinal tract that has immune protective effects and promotes colon health. By taking a probiotic combined with a sound nutritional eating plan you may be able to control some of those unwanted hormonal issues as well as all of the above. The community of microbes, or microbiome, outnumber our cells and have a100 fold more genes and enzymes capable of digesting food and regulating metabolism and immune health. It has been shown that disease often may correlate with a fall in the microbial diversity, so we could ask the question does disease cause a decline in microbial diversity or does a drop-in diversity cause or precede disease?

Evacuate -

Evacuation, or rather pooping is the final part of the digestive process. To aid and abet this scenario it would be wise if you are at all interested in either restoring health, prolonging your quality of life and preserving your age to supplement with a multi strain shelf stable probiotic to ensure bowel regularity. To repopulate healthy intestinal bacteria, we can choose a probiotic that can survive the stomach acid and bile production. One that supports the immune and digestive tract, relieves digestive complaints and promotes stool formation and excretion. Above all else, the major reason we are suffering from bowel complaints is that we are not moving enough to get rid of the junk from our trunk and not drinking enough plain ole water. Water helps in the elimination of waste products keeping the flow regular with ease. Slight changes are not that hard to implement. The hardest thing is to create the desire to make the changes, decide and commit. Even if you follow a protocol like Use it and lose it, move more and eat less everything becomes simple. It's basic, and not that complicated. We just over complicate it.

8

WHERE HAS OUR VILLAGE GONE?

After approaching health from a holistic point of view, I have determined that a great deal of health issues stem from a lack of personalisation, loneliness and love. Human connection is vitally important to personal health. My own family for example, although a little eccentric at times, has never lost the close connection and contact, despite our differences in geographical location, time zones and lifestyles. These interactions are threads of humanity which weaves in and out of our lives binding us together through communication and love. My family is a fortunate family that has experienced unfortunate circumstances, which family hasn't? But an important key to health and wellbeing is being surrounded by healthy, loving, supportive relationships. Susan Pinker, author

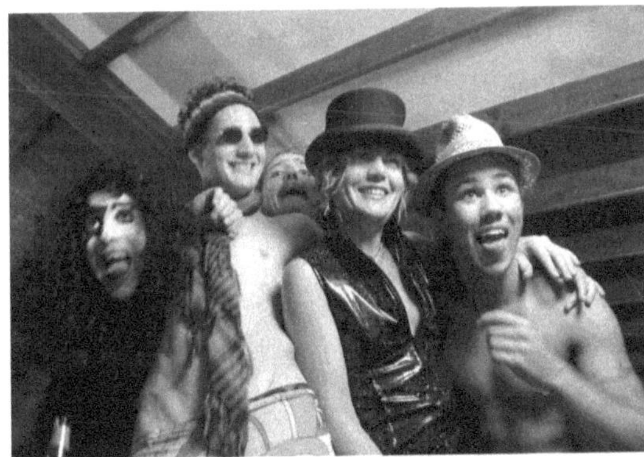

and social science columnist for *The Wall Street Journal* states that "Public isolation is the public health risk of our time". According to Susan Pinker, without positive relationships, people are more likely to be sick. Relationships do matter and are a stepping stone to health and longevity. People that live to a ripe old age of 100 and beyond, the centenarian's share a common thread. A life surrounded by family, friends, and a closely-knit community. The baker, the butcher, the local barista, they are never left to live solitary lifestyles. This differs greatly from our modern, mainstream world. (8) Two thirds of our world's population live in isolation and 80% of the world's population at some time or another will experience loneliness. It is a fact according to psychologist, Robert Waldinger, that people whom are socially connected to family, friends and community are happier, physically healthier and living longer. Through an intensive study of a group of 724 men from various walks of life over 75 years this was found to be true. (9)

Long gone are the days where the family would stay in the same town, take up the responsibilities of the family business and live within a couple of blocks from each other. The random occasional drop-ins from family and friends now correlate to a million texts to check if it is a suitable time to pop in for a 'cuppa' and a good old chin wag! Thirty years ago, when I lived in a small town of about 5000 people, everyone knew of the "sick" child that had just developed meningococcal. The whole town would rally together in support. The CWA, the 'Country Women's Association' would hone their baking skills and prepare cakes and biscuits to sell on the street corner to raise money for the family's medical payments. The family's school would hold a fete with other community organisations raffling off donations that would be given gladly from some of the meagre businesses that operated in the town. Currently, it is common to see so many people suffer loneliness and a trip to the doctor isn't necessarily because they are sick; they just want someone to talk to! Social relationships keep us happier and healthier, however loneliness kills. Loneliness is toxic, creating depression, declining health and declining brain function. The quality of relationships does matter!

They say it takes a whole village to raise a child. Whilst this is true, this doesn't seem to be the case today. The fact that there has been a huge shift away from our little towns to urban areas where work is more available, many families forsake familial ties in rural areas for career opportunities. In fact, so many relationships fail without the support of their close loved ones and live a life that is quite the opposite - a mediocre existence bereft of family support. What your grandparents had to put up with years ago for the sake of children is not the case these days. These days it seems to be more common for young girls to have babies regardless of social and financial circumstances. Perhaps our ideologies on the familial unit needs to be re-entrenched in society to reflect the close-knit communities and strong relationships our ancestors upheld. A child requires support, human interaction and nurturing from the moment they are born. Unfortunately, some of these values are lost in the modern world and some young parents remain focused on the social welfare cheque each week whilst sending their child to day care each day! Many millennials of our nation want everything now and are often not prepared to work towards the family unit, neglecting the wellbeing of their offspring to the point where welfare is wearing the brunt of their lack of conscious thinking. If you want to play grownups, this requires acceptance of the whole responsibility it takes to raise and nurture a child.

The amount of money our government spends on social welfare has created a deficit of billions of dollars which is ultimately being paid by other taxpayers! How does this action of enabling aid our society at large? We really are in trouble. People need to think about their actions and the consequences of them. For the sake of our children, for the sake of our family and for the sake of our society that appears to have lost all sense of values and morals. Progress once again, is not necessarily for the better of our society as it displays disadvantages in the development of our children. One may go as far as to say it contributes to the breakdown of the familial unit.

In a world that favours artificial intelligence and connectivity there has been an ever-increasing dysconnectivity and a shift away from personalisation. We live in a world where the art of engagement has been usurped by an apple (the iPhone, iPad, iPod, iTouch), technology and progress. Contrary to popular opinion, these devices are not necessarily making our lives simpler nor better on many levels! We are losing touch with what is real and meaningful to what is merely superficial! You only have to stop by your favourite coffee shop to see this. You can find the serious executive plodding into the café with earphones attached to his latest appendage, or a hipster swaggering in with his headphones glued to his well styled hair. The mother sitting restlessly in the middle of the café sporting the latest workout apparel juggles, shushes her loud demanding children yelling out for their baby-chinos whilst swooshing through the latest Instagram feed. Seriously? Yet, if we don't have it upon our person, it's like losing an appendage!! What did we do without them? Hey, I put my hand up and even I am guilty of that one! If I leave my own home without my iPhone I feel lost and out of this world. I think you know what I mean. I do not particularly like this phantom universal "inter-web of communication" however the positive intention of this device and the introduction of social media has turned sour. A great concept that was introduced to embrace communication to positively connect people, to unify, to further our knowledge and widen our experience, has opened a world full of unnecessary collisions between bad and good. This too has been a dilemma playing a part in the lost village concept. No-one speaks to anyone anymore, we just swipe right!!!!

Unfortunately, the art of conversation has been lost and overtaken through the new language of texting and social media. One of the predictors of living longer, healthier lives is having meaningful conversations and true social interactions with many people throughout your daily activities. It has been proven, that whilst you can use a phone, computer, or other technological device for communication, the individual is missing out on a whole cascade of neurotransmitters that are beneficial to the brain. When you engage with someone to converse on a one-on-one level, the eye contact through the speaking and listening process can omit a hormone, oxytocin, the 'love' hormone. This action within itself, can lower cortisol levels and thereby lessen stress. It is not entirely our fault as I don't think that we realise the serious health ramifications of our actions. We have lost the connectivity to real humans and forsaken this with artificial intelligence that seems to consume a great deal of time leading nowhere in particular!

Sean Parker, President of the social network Facebook had confessed that Facebook's goal was to "consume the conscious attention and time of the consumer". (10) Facebook and other social platforms have certainly changed the way humans are interacting. How does this sit within the context of health and wellbeing you may well ask? Well the response to that is that, this social media phenomenon has taken over our lives to the point where we now have social media addicts and mental health is synonymous with this epidemic. Users have become entrenched to the point that verbal communication is a thing of the past. Former Vice president Chamath Palihapitiya, admitted guilt when speaking to a group of graduates at Stanford, saying that they had created the tools that were ripping apart the social fabric of how society works! Melancholy, isolation, loneliness and depression have crept out of this network that set out with good intentions. Apparently, and according to Mr Palihapitiya, this has led to "moral discourse, non-cooperation, misinformation and mistruth".

Agghhh such is life, maybe I am old-fashioned and like social engagement via human contact. It's part of our social network and becomes extremely important as we age. Remember the centenarians! Communication via speaking, looking and touching may be the key to longevity in life. Having healthy supportive, loving relationships! No man is an island and communication and touch from human to human can save lives. If we become more aware, socially conscious and more loving then we can reach others. By doing one act of kindness, too can restore the step away from depersonalisation. Perhaps, we may have to rethink and raise our social consciousness to understand how negative this kind of progressive forward-thinking invention really is, may be its even time to put down the phone and do it alone!

9

HORMONAL HAVOC

Throughout our lives the ebb and flow of simple occurrences like hunger, emotions, blood sugar levels, acne, promiscuity, constipation, libido, fight or flight responses and metabolism can all be attributed to chemical messengers, neurotransmitters, or hormones. From the time we were born to the time we die; our body's communication system relies on both external and internal stimuli to aid even the most basic daily functions. This includes waking up, when to eat, when to stop, to how we think and even a quick response to an assault from a dog. Mental-pause, or otherwise known as menopause, adrenal dysfunction, polycystic ovarian syndrome, benign prostatic hyperplasia, diabetes are only just a few disorders due to hormonal mishaps. Welcome to the age of dysconnectivity. If a woman has heard it once she has heard it a thousand times. After screeching out through emotional pain and asking the question what the hell is wrong with me? The answer remains the same "it's probably your hormones". Before you go and stab me in the eyeball with your stiletto, (because of your histrionic outburst), pause, and consider .... am I right?

The real question is, what controls your hormones? The answer is nutrition ...... food ... full stop! Food provides the nutrients in your gut thereby regulating hormonal activity through natural biofeedback mechanisms. The brain is the Agency for central intelligence, or the other way around. It is the central intelligence agency that has a special unit, the pituitary gland. It responds to the physical body. The brain is not hard wired, as led to believe but more malleable to fire neurochemicals/ hormones to parts of the body that respond to action. We need energy for the brain to conduct the sophisticated symphony of minute messengers to sing their song in harmonic unison. The very food we eat can either break the link to these messengers or keep them connected so they can function optimally. Again, it all starts in the gut! Messages failing to function could mean disastrous results over time. If there is hormonal malfunction or dysfunction, chaos rules and there is no doubt that the amount of stuff pumped, inhaled, ingested or fed into your body will be responsible. It's like having a conversation with a blind-deaf person, they don't have a clue as to what is going on. Miscommunication can be a train crash waiting to happen!

These numerous and complex messengers profoundly affect the quality of our life, if not rule our life. A young male can expect a flood from a hormonal surge at the most inappropriate time just by looking at a young and very attractive female. Whilst on the other hand a premenstrual woman may stand there and cry. Normally, the calming neurotransmitters plays a role in balancing and controlling the other stimulating neurotransmitters. Low serotonin is one of the biggest causes of dysfunction and now a growing epidemic worldwide. In fact, Depression common in premenstrual women is due to the combination of low serotonin and oestrogen levels. Serotonin is considered 'the happy hormone', and a precursor to melatonin required for sleep and in turn defends against anxiety.

When serotonin is deficient that sense of mellowness that you once had turns into an overreactive insensitive dragon. Impatient, anti-social and just plain out of control. To top it off, whilst there is a decreased interest in normal activities there is an increased interest in carbohydrate and alcohol cravings which funnily enough feed this state. Once again, the monster within is unleashed and grows fervently in a state of heightened excitement.

And forget about patience, that went out the window along with sex!! Sound familiar? A visit, with a whinge and a whine, to your doctor can end up with a prescription of antidepressants. But as we already know, short term fixes do not boost serotonin production long term! Taking an anti-depressant prevents serotonin absorption, thereby lengthening its effect, so we have been told. A mediatory solution to perhaps a long-term problem. Have an apple, a chicken, an egg, or salmon or some other oily fish. Even better, if you are on edge go for a long walk, I mean a two-hour walk. Grounding yourself by getting in touch with the earth can make you happy and unhappiness is a breeding ground for disease Believe you me, these are by far better options, and there's a lot of truth in having an apple a day at keeping the Dr at bay!

If something ain't right, it is human nature to search for a solution. We have already discovered that a chemical to change biological energy is not the answer but here Food definitely can help. One essential amino acid called Tryptophan can assist in the production of serotonin. It is necessary for serotonin synthesis and can be found in dietary sources such as nuts, seeds, tofu, chicken, red meat, turkey, fish, oats, beans lentils and eggs!!! The recommended daily intake for tryptophan is 4mg per kilogram of body weight. When the diet is right, medicine is of no need. Remember, food first, then supplement. There is a supplement that raises serotonin levels to 5 HTP, which is naturally produced in the brain that begins with tryptophan. Once it is absorbed into the cell tryptophan is converted into 5 HTP the precursor to serotonin.

An article printed in an online journal Medicinetoday.com in March 2017 explained how diet effects depression with a correlation between nutrition and the microbiome in the GIT. A study performed at the Deakin university in Melbourne involved 56 patients with extraordinarily surprising results, revealing positive effects when using 5HTP on a group of depressive people. We know the answers, we provide the solutions, yet we still do not get it? Depression, mental illness, autoimmune disease, allergies, IBS, can all be attributed to miscommunication, deficiencies and imbalances. By addressing the imbalance with natural remedies such as food, water, sleep, love, vitamin and mineral therapy we too can survive to be well. It may be a long road, but we all make choices and we all choose a road, so we may as well choose the better one! Addressing hormonal communication and how they affect health is subject for another book being profound and integral for our wellbeing. In trying to mend broken pathways in order to avoid the 'train crash' we need to look at various macronutrients and lifestyle modifications to address this.

10

IS WATER THE FORGOTTEN MACRONUTRIENT?

"Water, water, everywhere, nor any drop to drink."
The rime of the ancient mariner. Samuel Taylor Coleridge.

Apart from the air we breathe, water is the most crucial element for sustaining life. We need water to survive and without it we would not. Without water, there is no life. All living animate objects that live in the animal and plant kingdom require water for critical bodily functions. Biochemical reactions, blood pressure, cellular hydration, respiration, metabolism, digestion, elimination and excretion of toxins all have one thing in common. They all require water. About 60-70% of your body's total mass is water and According to the Journal of Biological Chemistry, the brain and heart are composed of 73% water, lungs 83%, blood 80% and lean muscle 70%. (18)

The body needs more water than any other nutrient and is essential for life sustaining mechanisms including regulating body temperature, maintaining blood volume, electrical exchange and biochemical reactions. It is a nutrient carrier, major constituent of proteins, removes wastes and water participates in all metabolic activity. Unfortunately for us, water is an essential commodity that we not only *take for granted* but do not *take advantage* of. (18) Over the years water has been known to be a miracle cure for some very basic aliments including headaches joint pain and fatigue and most people do not realise that the quality of their structure, function and thought processes are dependent on the quantity and quality of water that they consume (or not consume)! (19)

With the abundant amounts of clear clean drinking water available in the western world you really must wonder why, in fact, we do not utilize this amazing elixir of life. Since many of our large water supplies have become contaminated, via treatment plants and recycling of wastes. Chemicals have been introduced in many metropolitan areas creating 'dead water'. Tap water, although treated with supposedly 'non-harmful' chemicals and toxins must be filtered, or our bodies will do this for us, via the kidneys or liver. Talk about busy, these organs never sleep! Is it any wonder that our filtration plant is really a dumping ground for "shit"? The liver is a sewerage system that is forever processing and getting rid of the junk from our trunk! Since water is 2 parts hydrogens, and 1-part oxygen, these chemicals have killed their molecular value making filtration an absolute necessity. Drinking boiled water, filtered water is our only option to gain the benefits of this powerful elixir.

Because of our shift from drinking water, toward large proportions of non-nutritional high caloric beverages, a higher prevalence of nutrition related diseases has emerged. Soft drinks like coca cola are mineral thieves not to mention a rust removalist. The elevated phosphates in these soft drinks leach vital minerals like magnesium, even propagating heart disease or osteoporosis from the lack of calcium. Mineral deficiencies can mean vitamin usage impairment. Chronic use and excessive amounts of soft drinks or sodas can lead to chronic elevation and depletion of glucose, leading to impaired insulin response furthering diabetes and promoting learning difficulties. Many soft drinks also contain aspartame which has been associated as being a cause of depression, insomnia and neurological disease. The pH of many soft drinks is about 2.5, enough to dissolve a 50-cent piece and incredibly 100 times more acidic than some of your organs. Disease, we have learnt thrives in an acidic environment and the sicker the person the lower the pH! So how does drinking water affect you? By just creating a habit of drinking water on a regular basis can improve productivity at work with improvement in concentration, keep you in shape and enhance your physical prowess.

Have you ever wondered why after an hour without any fluid the ability to think properly diminishes! A decline of only 2% of water can trigger short term memory loss and difficulty focusing. Although there is little evidence to prove this theory, studies performed by Benton & Burgess in children as young as 7 found that by drinking water enhanced their alertness, visual attention and memory. (20)

Water constitutes about 60% of an adult's body weight and a higher percentage in children. It makes common sense if we lose water we need to replace it. We know when we sweat, or perspire, as us women tend to prefer, water is lost to prevent overheating. When water alone is lost, ionic concentration increases therefore if you are a marathon runner or a tennis player or if you work long hours in the sun, you may get a sense that you need to ingest more salt. Whilst this has benefits, like replacing essential electrolytes lost, sometimes is it is better to drink plain old water. (20)

Water ingestion can lead to muscular fluidity and flexibility which alleviates cramps, lactic acid build up, prevents muscle strains and chronic injuries. Not drinking enough fluids can also lead to mild to moderate levels of dehydration. In studies conducted by Cian and colleague, findings include a loss of performance on short term memory creating confusion, disorientation, perceptual discrimination with arithmetic ability, visual-motor tracking and psychomotor skill. (20)

If you have ever had constipation, it is uncomfortable to say the least but by keeping well hydrated you can assist in elimination with little strain and more slide and glide. Water is the fluid that not only assists in the catabolic process of breaking down foods but also provides protection within the mucosal layer within your gastrointestinal tract.

Let's face it water is tasteless and for that matter less appealing than sweet fizzies. Try making water more palatable. Adding fresh cucumber slices assist the kidneys in elimination of impurities. An additional few mint leaves in water can ease the burden of nausea and the menthe tastes makes it a natural breath freshener or some coriander for a kick. A slice of lemon even though an acidic fruit can help your body to become alkaline, perfect for staying healthy. Disorders and diseases love an acidic state so if you choose to do one thing that will keep you well, do this one.

Apart from both fruit and vegetables being loaded with essential micro nutrients they contain a great deal of water. Watermelon and strawberries contain about 92 percent water per volume followed by grapefruit, cantaloupe, peaches, pineapple raspberries, cranberries and oranges holding 87 percent water by weight. Some high water by weight vegetables include broccoli cabbage, cauliflower, celery, cucumber, iceberg lettuce, sweet peppers, radishes, spinach, zucchini, and tomatoes. Is it any wonder why a nutritionist should suggest these vegetables if you want to lose weight? Loaded with water it is highly recommended that you eat about 9 servings every day according to Karen Collins, MS, RD, CDN, nutrition consultant to the American Institute for Cancer Research. I am not quite sure if that fits in with the original food pyramid and may look like a task too huge for most, but this equates to only about 2 ½ cups per day. (22)

Are you one of those people that sit with a plastic bottle at your desk and sip slowly through the day? Or do you have a bottle of water in your car that you take a swig whilst standing still at a traffic light? Well if you do, then it may be high time that you change this practice. Plastic bottles are made of a chemical called bisphenol

A, (BPA). BPA is a weak synthetic oestrogen called xeno-estrogen, found in many plastic products. These have been found to increase hormonal fluctuations in both men and women leading to hormonal driven cancers in both sexes. (23) BPA interacts with oestrogen receptors α and β, leading to changes in cell proliferation, apoptosis, or migration and thereby, contributing to cancer development and progression. (23) In 2002, clinical evidence found that these xeno-oestrogens initiate androgen-independent proliferation in human prostatic adenocarcinoma. (24)

In experimental studies in both humans and animals, BPA was originally thought to disrupt the oestrogen-triggered pathways by forming a transcriptional complex that can bind the oestrogen responsive element (ERE) in both antagonistic and agonistic mechanisms. The studies revealed that even at low doses BPA can induce oestrogen like activities in cells that are similar to oestrogen. (23,24). This is the danger, so choose your drinking vessel wisely and choose an excellent quality bottle or drink from glass.

How much is good enough?

There have been conflicting reports as to how much water we should drink each day. Roughly it is recommended by the better health campaign from the Victorian Government in Australia that women have approximately 2.1 litres p/d and men have about 2.6 litres p/d. From the official RDA website, it has been recommended that you drink 1 litre per 25 kg body weight. So, if you are about 49kg then you would drink just under 2 litres. (25)

Sometimes more is not necessarily better. Over drinking can cause hyponatraemia, depletion of the body's potassium stores. In extreme cases, drinking way too much leaving them in a catatonic state and sometimes death. Over hydration may be caused by water retention due to kidney disease, congestive heart failure, syndrome of inappropriate anti-diuretic hormone(SIADH). Prevention is always better than cure so stick to the rule of thumb of about 8 glasses, just like your grandmother told you years ago Your organs, skin and brain will love you for it in the long run.

It can be a pretty mean feat to get enough water but by following these simple practices you may improve your health. This is only a snapshot of the goodness that water has to provide, a smidgeon of a huge array of the benefits of drinking water, so grab a glass and sip throughout the day. By getting up from our computer to get another glass every 45 minutes could save you unwanted time in the gym sweating it out to lose those unwanted love handles. Doing this one simple task may alleviate headaches, improve your bodily functions, increase your exercise performance and lessen the effect of time.

11

PUT DOWN THE FORK AND WALK

As life rolls by, the speed of time seems to accelerate come midlife. As the clock ticks, changes march alongside us and for some these changes may be incremental but for some the effects of life with time can be devastating and life-altering. At the end of the day eliminate the emotional and spiritual criteria we are just' a machine'. A pump called the heart, is part of an efficient delivery system. It has a sophisticated arterial and venous network providing us with oxygenated blood, water and nutrients in around and out of the body. These networks are the connections that provide life. Oxygenation and micro vascularity is essential even to the far end of our peripheral regions like the tips of our fingers and tips of our toes. If these little vessels carrying oxygenated blood is even slightly impaired damage to the tissue can occur. Tissue damaging may cause blockages of blood triggering ischemia, a stroke or a heart attack.

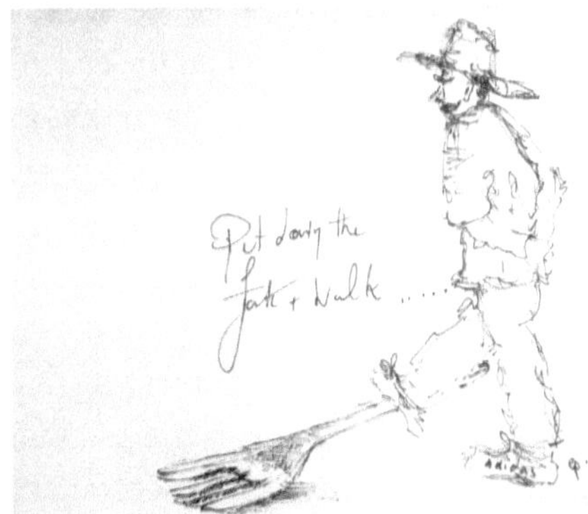

This machine, just like our cars needs to be fuelled, watered and oiled and lastly exercised. … Use it or lose it. When we age, muscle is lost by 2-3% every year beyond 40. After 40, your biological age speeds and can age faster than your chronological age. For every year that passes, you can age an extra 6 months. Meaning at the age of 49 you could literally be 53. Just wait till you hit your mid-50s, you can age up to 3 years for every 1. Something to look forward to, unless you move!

When we consider that we both use our body and car to get from A to B it is quite apparent that more time, energy and money is placed on our car rather than our body! This became evident when an old friend of mine helped me pour much needed oil into my worn-out Mazda, 'Elvis, (apparently, he's had" more hits than)!" Feeling rather ashamed as to how I care for him, it got me thinking that I was a poor host for my car. As I drove away from that worn-out man, I thought he was a pretty poor host to his body!! I guess it depends on your values and err …… Priorities! It also depends on how much you value your health, bottom line …………………… "there is no wealth without your health"!

> "Of all the courses which conspire to render the life of a man short and miserable, none have greater influence than the want of proper exercise"
>
> *18th century Scottish physician DR William Buchanan.*

For many years, we have been told to increase or add back the lost physical activity into our lives. We are creatures of comfort and habit and to change our routines is challenging. A clever "get off the couch" program called "Life be in it" was introduced in Australia in the 70s via a couch potato character called "Norm". Norm did his best to sell the concept of moving more for our health. Having some benefit for a while, we lost it and have adopted other distractive sedentary practices instead. In an article in the Courier Mail in 2015, the message was loud and clear coming from a concerned Health Minister at that time, Sussan Ley urging all Australians to "put down the remote" and "go for a walk". The article revealed that one in five Australians has at least two chronic diseases brought on by obesity, smoking and inactive lifestyles – including heart or lung disease, arthritis and back problems, (statistics provided by the Australian Institute of Health and Welfare). I understand that this is not a new concept and We have all heard this message time and time again, but is any one listening?

We are not designed to sit behind a desk squashing our liver. We are not designed to stare at glaringly-bright-lit up screen for eight hours, each day, five days a week. What happened to the days of real physical activity when cars were less, and bikes were the norm. We used our god given legs to walk everywhere. This is not rocket science, this is simple, old fashioned and basic. Whenever I trained a client in the gym and they couldn't quite get the hang of it, I thought of an old saying that a mentor used to say to make things simpler, 'get back to the stick.' In other words, going back to basics and omitting other unnecessary stuff.

"Exercise thy casting youth defends"

Arnold Schwarzenegger, philanthropist and former Governor of California is probably better known for his contribution to professional bodybuilding. Widely considered to be among the greatest bodybuilders of all time as well as bodybuilding's biggest icon and having one of the best well put together bodies of all time (my thoughts actually !!), his movie 'Pumping Iron', compares body building to having sex. It is an interesting take on weight bearing exercise. He describes the associated pleasure flooding his body whilst performing contractions, like the peak of his sexual experience. It was the release of the movement as though it was the crescendo or the climax of sex. That should be enough to entice us to move more and get back into the gym! Surely!!!

One of the best type of training that you can add to your existing health regime is endurance training. It is by far the best way to protect the body's metabolism from the effects of aging. The side effects are positive. A huge compilation of effects from moving effortlessly like a reduction of body fat, increased sensitivity to

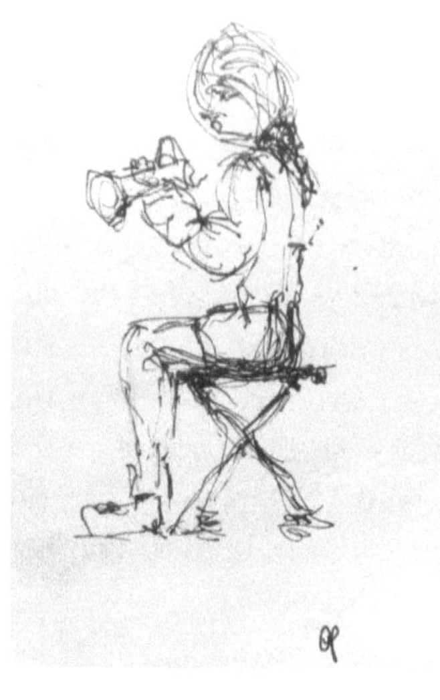

insulin, thereby decreasing risk of diabetes and other metabolic disorders like thyroid function. Increasing lean body mass increases testosterone, boost HDL levels, lowers LDL levels, improves neurological communication, boosts mood enhancing hormones like GABBA, dopamine and serotonin. The changes that physiologists attribute to aging are caused by disuse and using your body with endurance type resistance training and a certain type of long distance walking will keep your body young.

Before everyone freaks out and think that I am suggesting they train like a marathon runner, (if you want to go out on the road and flog yourself by all means but this will increase the oxidative process). It is merely the longer and slower walks that I recommend.

One of the secrets of ridding 'the junk from the trunk' is to stay mobile and fluid. I know I harp on this one concept but I've used this concept many times and it works. Walk like a Victoria Secret model (without the swagger)! Get in touch with the ground and feel connected to every part of your anatomy. Stand tall with correct posture as your spine realigns, so will your organs. Everything becomes more efficient. Oxygen pumps away evenly and not at a neurotic state. Pent up stress disperses, dissolving away naturally. At the very least, like most of my clients, expect a better mood, glowing skin and fat loss! The best thing about this new type of walking is that it costs nothing and involves only one thing. Action. At any age put down the fork and walk will get rid of your junk from your trunk!

12

GET RID OF THE JUNK FROM YOUR TRUNK

"Energy can neither be created nor destroyed……..
only transferred."

Einstein

Just imagine for a minute that you are at a cocktail party. The champagne, Verve, Bollinger is flowing! Effervescent and light, you take a sip and continue until the bubbles fill your head making you giddy with delight. The rather easy on the eye, well put together male waiter attempts to alter the consistency of this fine delicacy by topping up your crystal glass. As he pours the champagne into the existing glass the bubbles lose their original appeal and the result is only half the effect. To get the original effect of the amazing drop is to drink all of it first and then have a completely fresh one. This is why we need to walk coolly and slowly, to completely deplete the old energy from the cell before we can add any new energy requiring substrates. Get rid of the junk from your trunk, takes on a whole new meaning. Use the existing energy first and then start the process all over again with good fuel ………………… Nutrition!

Same goes with the concept of resistance training. Anti-aging strategies, means slowing your biological age below your chronological age. Endurance resistance training extends beyond heavy weights, short bursts of high impact activity and 2 – 3 rep type sets. Longer periods of cortisol and insulin releasing type of endurance training will get rid of the junk from your trunk, help you to calm down and not wind you up!! Resistance enhances muscle mass, strength and preservation of cartilage and bone and could be the difference between getting osteoporosis or not! What and how we trained in our 20s just doesn't cut it in our 4th, 5th, 6th decade and beyond. We just don't get the same results that we got way back then.

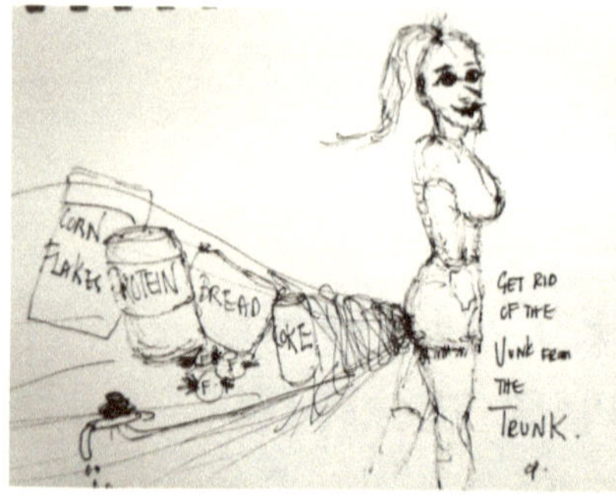

The food we eat everyday will supply us with nutrients that we need or don't need. But we already know that, yet, our actions do not correlate with this at all. It is not, about calorie counting or eating less to shift weight but a great deal more. It is complex yet very simple. The major problem is that we are not releasing our energy in the right way. Many health experts have always advocated releasing energy by mainly two ways evacuation and through respiration (predominately cardio). Energy, if not cleared can accumulate and usually as we look down to our naval it is the accumulation over the playground that becomes the major concern for our health and our life expectancy. Funnily enough if you are physically moving and engaged, then it is more likely that you will feel more mentally energised and engaged! We need to not only move more but provide only the energy that we require to perform our daily functions it is not about getting puffed but, a cycle of depletion that is far more important.

If energy can be transferred, we just have to think of a block of ice. It is just water that is frozen. If we apply heat it will change to a liquid, apply a bit more heat and it changes from a liquid to a gas, like fat. At first, the fat may be as hard as a rock We increase the heat, get rid of the junk from the trunk (stop eating as much) increase movement to create the heat, and voila, fat just like the ice cube melts, then suddenly disappears. This does happen over time yet requires effort, energy, action, persistence and patience! Getting to your set point or what is termed desired weight and packing on some muscle will set you in good stead for the future. Muscle is more efficient at utilising calories whilst excessive fat is not. And in the words of Homer Simpson .... Doh!

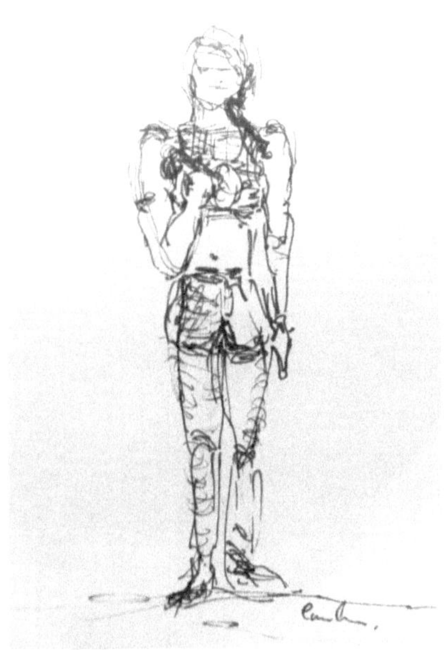

13

IS THE DAIRY GONE FROM OUR DAIRY?

Out of interest and curiosity, I searched the inter-web for information regarding the nutritional value of dairy. OMG, holy cow! There are countless articles that are headed with statements like, *the truth about milk; You may never drink milk again; 5 ridiculous myths about cow's milk; Should humans drink cow's milk?* and *12 frightening facts about milk.* On the one hand this is presented to us loud and clear,

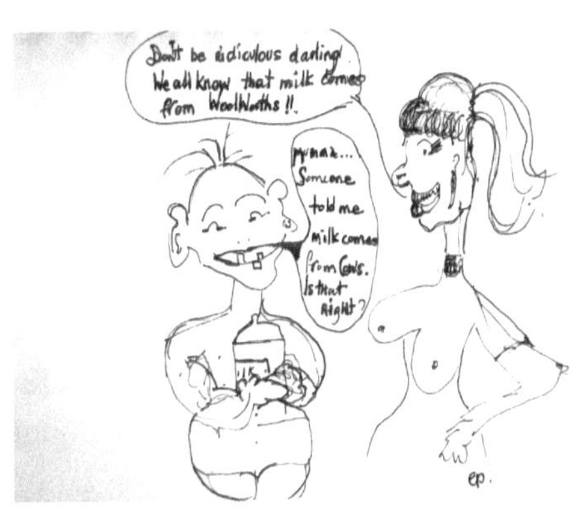

but on the other hand milk is still used widely and even presented as having health benefits. Who doesn't love a thick shake or a good old-fashioned ice-cream. Milk and other dairy products are good for us, so we have been told … where else does our calcium come from? Cow's milk is not the only source of calcium and is not a recommendation based on strict science. There are many other alternatives providing us with our recommended daily intake or RDI. Perhaps in another decade it may have been, but presently, this is not the case. Unfortunately, there is contradictory information available which creates confusion about this topic. Alternate practitioners advocate that milk is pro-inflammatory and according to Dr Hyman (integrated medical DR). Going as far to say, "Dairy *is* nature's perfect food — but only if you're a calf". (28) The fact of the matter is that the advanced practices of homogenization and pasteurization has interfered with what used to be natural liquid gold to what now may be considered as a major health risk! Since pasteurization and homogenization, we have lost the nutritional quality of milk. To be fair to the cow, it may not necessarily be only the milk that is unhealthier, but other additives combined with the milk to alter its taste that are the villains. Caramel and chocolate toppings, lashings of sugar upon additives make these treats a hyperactive nightmare for any parent. What happened to plain old water?

The process of 'cleaning' milk involves heating denaturing the proteins available in milk. This process destroys vital enzymes including lactase, making it difficult for lactose to be digested properly. Lactose is the sugary part of milk and since these vital enzymes capacity of conversion has been lost the lactose builds up in the system. Accumulation from excessive amounts can keep you farting and starting, bloating and belching, from breakfast to tea! Conventional cow's milk has also been known to be associated with leaky gut, thanks to the pasteurization process and the A1 casein-protein present. It is not a news flash that calcium is required for bone strength and teeth formation, but calcium also influences hormonal function, muscular and blood vessel function nerve signalling and blood clotting. Unfortunately, the heat of these processes also kills the Vitamin C and other minerals that generally support the bone matrix which are naturally present in raw milk. The Pasteurization process alters calcium into another form, difficult for absorption. Denaturing also destroys little of the naturally occurring iodine. Iodine, a trace mineral stored in the thyroid gland is essential to metabolic function and the driver of growth. It role is vital in the process of growth and early development of all organs, particularly the brain. Iodine deficiencies, have led to cognitive decline in children and according to the World health organisation "it is the most prevalent and easily preventable case of impaired cognitive development in children in the world"'.

Young mothers, concerned for their children's teeth development are worried that the lack of milk consumption will hinder their growth and strength. As I observe their little faces and bodies and take note of their mannerisms, for most part of the time, IF the child ate more fruit and vegetables they wouldn't need to worry. Apart from calcium, they would get loads of essential minerals, plus the fighter nutrients (phytonutrients) that could aid their immune system and development. Yet they avoid them like the plague (28) For whatever reason vegetables at a young age is an acquired taste. When I was young we were forced to eat our greens and those disgusting Brussel sprouts and squishy peas before we left the table or had dessert. Mind you I believe I had my fair share of making a huge mish mash of green mess on the floor of the local RSL club on our once in a blue moon dining out experience! Peas somehow found their way into other cavities in my body for amusement to the extreme that one got stuck in my nose for hours. Never the less, we did eat them and if we did not we would starve. Call me old fashioned, but taste is an acquired one. Convenience is another and sometimes we offer the children food according to our taste!

Snotty noses and another antibiotic

If you and your children have ever been so lucky as to have a green nose, then there is no doubt that there may be an infection. We can play the blame game as to where did it eventuate but in many cases that snotty nose is purely from drinking too much milk! Dairy products create mucous which seem to accumulate in the nasal cavities under our eye sockets. Small children that drink mostly milk as their staple, end up being, clogged in these areas leading to inflammation or infection. Ears, nose and throat infections associated with mucous overload and bacterial infections may be purely reliant on milk. It is also common that drinking milk can lead to bacterial overgrowth in the digestive tract, affecting the gut microbial diversity in turn, affecting both the immune system and the brain. It does not come as a surprise that there is a link between children on the autistic spectrum and drinking too much milk. These little ones, may experience symptoms like hyperactivity, irritability, loose bowels, constipation, impulsivity, excessive dribbling and an inability to focus from this excessive mucous. Although there is a temptation to go far as to say that we have become an age of "autism', with that term being used rather loosely. By eliminating this one food group I have seen those little children have remarkable 'cures' from this affliction. As the child is weaned from the bottle and with age the Eustachian tube, from ear to nose, widens and becomes more diagonal in shape lessening the load. This means there are fewer blockages, less infections to both inner and outer ear, nose and even throat. (30) A client exclaimed her amazement about how both her daughter's behaviour and health improved out of sight by eliminating all dairy plus gluten after only one week of doing so. Her eyes shone brightly as she marvelled at the changes. By changing from plain cow's milk to a nut milk has made life more bearable for not only the children but the mum as well. If you have doubts, then experiment and see.

It is not only the children that are affected by milk. Since we have become a café society, and 'ladies who like to lunch', the odd latte, cappuccino or skinny flat white based on pasteurised normal milk may be ok on the odd occasion, but not every day which seems to be the norm. This may be enough to deregulate your gut, cause pain, irritability, constipation and internal corruption. And we wonder why we are fat? The pasteurisation process converts the lactose into another form, called beta lactose, which is rapidly absorbed and may adversely raise blood glucose levels. (30) Having other options can be helpful so if you are out and about and need a social hit. Make other choices. Try a green smoothie with a chlorella, kale, rocket and apple, with half a banana and coconut water. Or create your own using coconut options, celery, cucumber, pineapple, chia seeds, parsley, mint and flaxseed oil. These foods combined will give you more bang for your buck supplying one third of the protein needed by an average adult with cleansing and alkalising effects upon the body.

Other dairy products that have stood the test of time containing nutritious benefits are raw milk, A2 cow's milk, goats, sheep, camel and buffalo milk. Coffee also robs the body of much needed calcium and by sitting in the sun sipping on a latte in the morning may be good for two reasons. Sunlight assists our body to synthesise vitamin D which seems to be deficient in 80% of the western world's population and has been correlated to thyroid dysfunction, obesity, osteoporosis and cancer. Being a pro hormone, it assists calcium to be absorbed into the much-needed bone. Be careful of supplementing with calcium alone as it should be taken with vitamin D 3 along with K2, (menaquinone) making bones more flexible and less likely to break. Every woman over 50 should be using these three nutrients in the correct formulations.

If you are in menopause, you may be deficient and a likely candidate for osteoporosis. The long and the short of it either limit your cow's products or swap your cow's milk with other plant-based milks. You will thank me for that later.

14

BALANCE THE pH FACTOR.

Balancing our body's acid to base level seems to be more challenging these days particularly since we have a misconception as to what we are attempting to balance. Our body's acid alkaline balance is known as its pH balance. Measured on a scale from 0-14 with 0 being highly acidic and 14 being highly alkaline. Clinical trials have proved that an alkaline body is much healthier than an acidic body, however various organs *need to be more alkaline and less acidic* and *some more acidic than alkaline.* When we talk about pH it really should be in reference to our blood which optimally should be between 7.2 and 7.45. Nearly all of my patients are too interested in alkalising, yet I don't think they fully understand that we have to have a balance within our system so that each organ can function optimally.

The acidic environment in your digestive tract, stomach and intestines is hugely important, as this is your first line of defence against pathogens that enter your digestive system. The stomach has the highest acidity level in the human body. Its pH level is between 2-4 to dissemble foods and is strong enough to disintegrate a coke can! The colon, part of the digestive tract requires a slightly less acidic environment a pH between 5.5 and 7. Candida albicans an opportunistic fungus (or form of yeast) prefers an alkaline environment and assists in reducing the acidity within the intestines.

Those rather embarrassing blurts of sulphur wafts may be caused by one of the by-products, ammonia, formed from the yeast fermentation of sugar. This concurrently increases the alkalinity of the digestive tract and promotes other yeasts growth. We all have probably felt the difference.

A man around the age of 36 recently asked for my help as he felt he was too acidic. Learning that he had rather an active social life, with a huge intake of alcohol, it was no wonder that he felt inflamed bloated and acidic. It was not uncommon for him to drink half a bottle of vodka after several bottles of a good quality red, a few nights per week. Adamant that he was not going to change, all I could do was introduce some much-needed positive suggestions to assist the process of removing the unwanted acids and support his liver. Apple cider vinegar, activated B vitamins, Vitamin C and a herbal mixture of liver enhancing properties were prescribed. As far as I know, whilst he was especially grateful for my advice he is still waddling around health food stores, chafing his thighs, shuffling to the nearest apple cider vinegar aisle, combining it with garcinia cambogia, as someone had announced on Facebook that it is the latest alkaline and weight loss promoting trick (without doing anything physical … Seriously???) Get with the program, get off the couch take a walk and put down the fork!!! An acid body generally gives rise and supports cancer growth. It is preferable that we have about 70-80% of alkaline forming foods in our diet and 20-30% of acid forming foods but for most of us, this is more likely the reverse.

Metabolic acidosis is a condition in which the body produces too much acid or when the kidneys cannot remove or neutralise acids in the body and is extremely dangerous. Scientists have found that low grade chronic metabolic acidosis is common but often goes undetected because it most often occurs despite normal blood pH and bicarbonate levels. Fad diets and advertised diets that advocate life sustaining properties may in fact be highly acidic and long term can cause kidney and liver damage that can be fatal. To avoid this inflammatory state, it is a better option to choose colourful life enhancing fresh vegetables, stay away from fads and eat easy to digest proteins. Never eat the same meal twice in a row, change it up, watch your portions, frequency and combinations. Drink more water and keep it simple, when we complicate it, "it", then becomes complicated.

High alkaline forming foods

Leafy greens, avocados, celery, kale, rocket, spinach grapefruit, cucumber, grapes, kiwi fruit, TOMATO, bokchoy, apple cider vinegar, coconut cider vinegar, soy, almonds, lemon, limes melons strawberries and many other fruits, wheat grass, chia seeds, chlorella.

High acid forming foods

Animal proteins, including beef, lamb, port, chicken shellfish, duck eggs & dairy refined cereals, sugar fizzy drinks including coke, lemonade, alcohol & processed foods.

15

CALM YOUR FARM

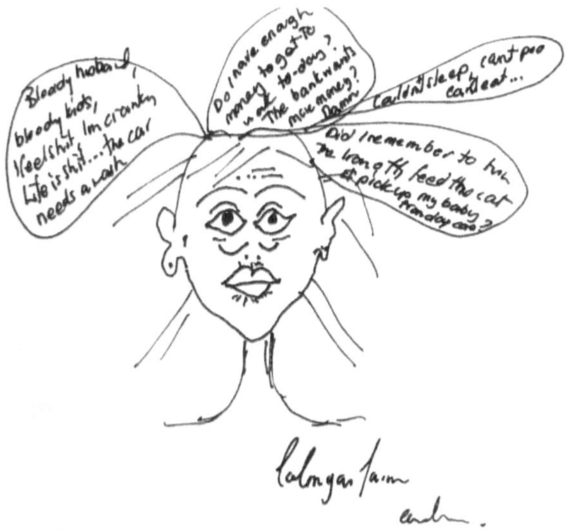

I was walking with one of my clients on the beach one day when she asked me if it was normal that if she woke up in a bad mood, the whole house would become affected and they too would be in a bad mood? That, you could guarantee. I sniggered at that question. She was right. My mind flicked back to the times that I was over tired and stressed. Juggling work as a photographer, an artist an athlete, a mother and a wife, life was full-on, finding myself little time to calm down. The disproportionate amount of energy consumed by daily living sucks your vital energy and leaves you with minimal amount to spend on the things that actually-matter, which is Your family and your health. Even if the other house dwellers woke feeling bright and breezy, suddenly their whole energy level changed according to yours, effecting *their* mood. But the mouse on the wheel continues to swiftly move until he drags his feet over the hard wire on the wheel until he, stumbles and, well, falls off his perch. Sound familiar? What are the mice in search of anyway? What's the point again; remind me? What is **it** that zaps our energy? Life's continual demands? Or is it a simple thing as being aware of your energy levels and the lack thereof.

In the here and now, it is the stresses that we place on yourself in our life created through the dictations of society. We demand it, or we allow the doctrine of society to dictate what we should be, have or want. Without a doubt stress is the most debilitating emotion caused from fear. Fear of what? The more we do, the more we have and then so it seems the more we want. Until one day eventually you realise you cannot get blood out of a stone! You wear out or you wear down.

Stress can be one of those environmental stimuli's causing inflammation. Most illnesses begin with stress producing thoughts creating tightness or strain within our bodies. The tension created within our body has the propensity to lower our immunity. Our subconscious minds, tends to lower our defence mechanisms in response to stress, suppressing our natural immune response and therefore we are more prone to illness. Prostaglandins are potent lipid mediators that increase blood flow, summon white blood cells moving swiftly through the body to remove possible antigens or nasty pathogens. This is a natural response to defend the body, however the prostaglandin overactivity can play an emerging role in cancer progression.

These inflammatory pathways may be activated by the foods we eat, the thoughts we think, infectious agents, irradiation and other environmental stimuli. Financial burden and relationships play a key role in having a major effect on the body contributing to an over production of cortisol and the other adrenal chemical messengers trying to adapt to the constant threats of modern life. These prostaglandins account for 95% of all cancers with Survival and proliferation of cancer stem-cells appearing to be dependent on the activation of these inflammatory pathways.

No matter what way you look at it, disease is Inflammation. Inflammation, so it seems, is the main driver of all chronic disease. This weakened state can increase your risk of many diseases starting with anything that has an "itis" on the end of it. Pancreatitis, can lead to pancreatic cancer, cystitis can lead to kidney or other urological cancers, fibro-cystitis of the breasts can lead to cancer. I eat well, says poor Norma, who looks like she has swallowed a spare tyre. "but I just can't budge the weight"! Poor Norma, has been eating according to her version of 'healthy', for quite some time now. Adopted many dietary fads borrowed from the internet given to thousands of people in their 50s, suffers from hormonal hell, stressed to the max, hates her husband, never drinks alcohol and never has sex! Where's the love? Norma, is a modern-day version, of what I term, 'running from the lions'. Norma, lives in a fear-based world as opposed to a love based one. Norma is the norm and is synonymous with 80% of the western world's population living in this state … and living in this state can make you seriously fat or seriously ill.

Being over-weight doesn't always come from over-eating, but it could be from chronic stress endured over time and throughout our lives lowering our basic function of digestion. The question is, do we create the stress and then endure the stress? Chronic stress plays a huge role in the inflammatory process. According to American practicing chiropractor Dr Eric Berg, stress creates more *alkalinity* in our digestive organs, impairing their functions. One of these organs is the gallbladder and its role is to emulsify fats that we obtain from our diet. If this role is compromised a layer of fat can hang over your belt, as attractive as it may be, it is usually called a muffin top! The substance bile is produced by hepatocytes in the liver and stored in the gall bladder, comprised of bile salts, cholesterol, potassium, sodium and pigments from the breakdown of haem (red blood cells.) Our bodies synthesize about 1 cup of bile every day which is constantly drip fed into the liver. When we have this organ removed, it usually makes it difficult for weight loss and weight even harder to regulate. When a surgeon rips out that organ for whatever reason, and in some cases, when it is absolutely necessary, it may have fixed one problem, but weight gain can be another problem affecting not only your body but your mind. Turmeric is one nutrient that aids in bile production and regulation. Turmeric may also reduce bloating caused by indigestion or dyspepsia. It is also a powerful anti-oxidant, as powerful as Vitamin E and Vitamin C and it creates enzymatic activity in the liver preventing toxic overload. Radical surgery causes inflammation to promote healing. Inflammation whilst being warranted, may also leave you susceptible to a bacterial or viral infection. A lowered immune response may increase a general feeling of malaise; therefore, you don't feel like eating, your thought patterns become scattered with a decline in vitality, and naturally your health. In a warped and twisted sense, you actually need to be well to afford the luxury of being sick. A double-edged sword scenario.

16

LET'S GET BACK TO MOTHER NATURE - MACRONUTRIENTS.

So where to now? I guess we really should understand the macro nutrients that we require to optimise bodily functions. There are three main substrates called macronutrients that make up our food. These macronutrients are classified as protein, carbohydrates and fats. The most exciting part about these, that in their natural state they can restore vital properties relating to the mind body and spirit. Have you ever experienced the queasiness after eating a Big Mac or after gorging on your mother's favourite macaroni and chunky potato salad, slathered in a pool of mayonnaise made from condensed milk? I expect the feeling is not great. If you eat heavy, you will be heavy, if you eat light and fresh, you guessed it, you will be light. The following pages are dedicated to give you a better understanding about their role and their effects on how we think, feel and perform. In a rat race world of being busy and convenience, getting it right could halve your risk of having any disfunction or disease.

That old saying, you are what you eat is unquestionably true. Great attention is given to the foods we use to nourish and sustain our bodies, but equally important, is the combinations of macronutrients, the portions and the frequency of eating that counts. The foods that we eat create energy and fresh fruits and vegetables, whole grains, legumes, seeds and nuts, easily digestible proteins are preferable choices over hamburgers, fried foods, and donuts, pizzas and pastas. The latter bogs you down, whilst the former are nourishing foods for not only the body, but the soul. Everything that you put into your mouth influences your body which then effects your brain, your mind and your emotions!

It all starts, even before a babe leaves the womb and enters the world. From mother to child, the baby is fed through the umbilical cord. We now know, thanks to science, that if the immune system of the host, the mother, is compromised at that time, then more than likely the child's immune system will be too. The highest quality foods are contained in natural living foods. Amino acids, minerals and vitamins are in their finest forms from energy enhancing carbohydrates, body building protein and anti- inflammatory fats with the correct amount of trace elements, oxygen, enzymes and hormones found naturally in nature.

Dr. Minnach, a functional medicinal practitioner, Ph.D. in Medical Sciences (holistic nutritionist) believes that both the body and soul are intimately connected to the food we eat. She believes that food nourishes much more than just our bodies, nurturing both body and soul. The more 'alive' food is the better it is for us due to its active constituents. Dr Hyman, functional Medical physician and founder of the functional medicine unit in USA says that there is no such thing as junk food. There is only junk and food.

Fascinating biochemistry, provide the rationale to not only theories, but countless real-life evidence-based data to indicate that the nutrients gained from food can shift stagnant energies in relationship to the physical and psychological being and thereby the spiritual outlook in one's life. (27) All Food has energetic values measured in glycaemic values. Sugars and other carbohydrates like potatoes have a higher glycaemic value. Fat too is termed as being highly caloric but is not necessarily the evil villain as once thought. Who ever invented the no fat, low fat diet was probably one of the worst dieticians or so-called health expert ever. Essential fatty acids are needed and act, not only as insulation, has a role in hormone synthesis and the capacity to modulate inflammation. Whether you choose good or bad options, food has the capacity to alter not only the way you look but the way you think and the way you feel.

The staple diet of our illustrious land down under is based on Poly sugar combinations with man-made fats. Men sing songs about a vegemite sandwich, meat pies, kangaroos, bangers and mash. Our good old barb-i with bangers on bread smothered with tomato sauce is not a barbie without them! These foods are primarily sugar. Too much has more potential to create the love handles that will not budge. Too much sugar produces more glucose needed to be pumped into the cell. Too much sugar, like anything can be harmful and leads to an insensitivity to glucose. De-sensitivity to the hormone insulin, means that glucose has a hard time to move from the liver to the muscle, gets stored in the liver as glycogen and waits for energy expenditure. Whilst you choose to lay on the couch or sit in your arm chair knitting, the energy, is then stored as, you guessed it, fat!

I was taken aback recently when a young girl asked if we had any sugar-free maple syrup. She was on a low-carb-sugar-free diet and had read a book about being sugar free. The poor girl was embarrassed and looked confused when my colleague and I stared back at her totally perplexed. Apparently, she had been advised from some so-called health expert that this option was a better alternative to sugar. Surprised? I guess I shouldn't be. Maple syrup is predominately sucrose, which is common table sugar which is a naturally occurring disaccharide and found in the sap of the maple tree. It is not sugar free.

17

DREAD OR FEAR CARBS!?.........
DAMMED IF WE DO AND
DAMMED IF WE DONT

"Sugar how you get so high, if you get burned then
don't be surprised"

Robyn Shultz

What are carbohydrates and why do we need them? Carbohydrates
Include sugars, glycogen starches and cellulose. Even though they
are a large and diverse group of organic compounds and have several
functions, carbohydrates represent only 2-3 % of your total body
mass. Carbon, hydrogen and oxygen are the elements found in
carbohydrates of which the ratio of hydrogen to oxygen atoms is
usually 2:1. The same as in water. Carbohydrates generally contain
one water molecule for each carbon atom, this is the reason they
are called carbohydrates which means watered-carbon. The three
groups of carbohydrates based on their sizes are monosaccharides,
disaccharides, and polysaccharides.

In humans, carbohydrates function mainly as a source of chemical
energy for generating Adenosine Tri-Phosphate(ATP), needed to
drive metabolic reactions. From inching over the line of a marathon,

to utilising brain energy for an exam, carbohydrates provide this energy. Only a few carbohydrates are used for building structural units. One example is Deoxyribose, a type of sugar found in ribose, a building block for deoxyribonucleic acid (DNA), your genetic blueprint. This molecule carries genetic information requiring certain nutrients, specifically the B vitamins, particularly B12, for correct cellular replication.

If the whole point of eating is for energy, then where do we get our energy from? A carbohydrate is just one of the substrates that yield energy in the form of sugars. Every piece of food that we eat yields a different amount of energy and carbohydrates provide sugars that convert to glucose indicated by a glycaemic index (GI). Many foods although not seen as sugar will convert to glucose. A client of mine told me one day that he needed to "get his health back on track' as his weight had escalated out of proportion as he did not feel at all well. As he sat with me and woofed down his eggs, bacon and toast he told me that he does not have sugar. I asked him what he had eaten for the last few days. His diet had included a lot of beer, wine, gluten free bread, some Thai and Indian cuisine and fruit. Most of these foods, I explained, are carbohydrates that are converted to glucose, simply put, they are sugar. Just because you do not have table sugar in your tea, coffee or sprinkled on Weetabix, you are still consuming these foods that will break down to the smallest unit of sugar. I am still surprised to hear that people think that rice, potatoes and bread are _the only carbohydrates_ and neglect the fact, that carbs are represented in various forms including our most needed fruit and vegetables.

Whilst some people obviously do not care about the composition of food, many carbohydrates present tremendous fear, especially to those who seek the perfection in body, shape or a desirable form. This mishap has led to confusion as to what to eat, how much to eat, when to eat and why do we eat them at all. A lettuce leaf is a carbohydrate, so is a tomato as well as other fruit, vegetables, rice, pasta, breads, cakes, biscuits and sweets. I see, only too often people in search of a natural protein bar with a low-carb content. Being overly concerned about the amount of carbs, they overlook the high sodium content and other synthetic substitutes in that bar. Even though clearly labelled, they are unrecognised and problematic for our bodies. If its manmade it is unnatural, yet eating the real deal, like wholesome fruit such as an apple or a banana incites a world of fear due to high fructose content. The major difference is that fruit contain a multitude of energy creating nutrients, fibre and minerals that act as spark plugs moving this machinery, inside and out! A lot of fruits ranked as "dangerous" contain polyphenols, chemical based molecules that act as antioxidants. These are the phyto-nutrients, having disease protective mechanisms and as I said earlier, the fighter nutrients. Some vegetables contain cellulose, the fibrous carbohydrate providing necessary vitamins and extra bulk for optimal digestion and elimination.

Today's western diet promotes high carbohydrate laden foods which convert to glucose triggering insulin to be released from the pancreas. After a while this organ gets hammered and tired of reacting to the amounts of sugar being pumped into the body. This enormous stress placed on this organ may weaken and desensitised to respond to glucose. As a result, we are seeing an increase in what we call metabolic–X–syndrome, a predisposition to diabetes 2. The constant use of this organ often sets our internal environment for other diseases to develop, including cancer. The type and the amount of carbohydrates you consume affects your blood sugar levels. The largest rise in blood sugar occurs from … surprise, surprise …… vegetables, followed by breakfast cereals, biscuits, fruit, dairy products and lastly dried legumes. Somewhat surprising, as you would not really expect vegetables in the form of carrots, parsnips and potatoes to send your glucose response soaring, but these do. However, we usually eat these vegetables cooked and with other substrates as in the old Sunday roast, or stir fry's and stews. Obviously, anyone that is considering weight control, and or are diabetic, need to focus on other factors to manage the highs and lows of insulin response. Portion control and choosing wisely can save you a dance with diabetes as negative carbohydrate laden food create an insulin response leading to a rise and fall of glucose and a need for more. Having protein and fat with carbohydrates slow down the insulin response providing satiety and a sense of energy for a longer period.

Consider for one second you are sitting around a campfire. The fire is burning a little low, to keep the flames burning brightly the fire needs to be stoked and fuel is required. Imagine that carbohydrates are the paper that you place on this fire. The paper will burn brightly, but for only a few seconds. You then place a few twigs or sticks on the fire to keep it going, knowing that you really need to put a whole log on, so you do not have to get up again so quickly. The twigs and sticks are the protein that you ingest, and the logs represent the fat in your diet. It is the combination that hold you in good stead to provide you with the energy that you require and so that you can perform various functions without an energy deficit daily. To sustain daily functions, you also need to consider, whether you are eating whole fruit, or drinking the juice of the fruit, whether food is cooked or uncooked, whether we eat it with a meal containing trans-fat, the amount of protein and whether or not fibre is associated with it, all of these factors influence the rate of the rise and peak level of blood sugar. The rise and fall of the flames!

Glucose is the main fuel for the body cells. Fructose participates in metabolism. Galactose is found in erythrocytes of individuals with B-type of blood. Sugar has been labelled "the white death" and is one of the most addictive substance on the planet. Eating too much sugar in any of its forms will make you fat, and sugar is sugar no matter what form it comes, whilst sugars in whole fruit and vegetables promote health others decrease health, promoting disease! For this very reason, _most_ nutritionists focus more on a higher proportion of vegetables compared to fruit in the diet. True, advocating a fruit free diet is eliminating natural fructose yet we are eliminating wholesome food that outweigh the negative effect due to the high amount of essential minerals and vitamins they contain. Berries, bananas, kiwi fruit and the odd apple or two will not kill you and in fact may just save your life. Try eating more onions to lower your blood sugar while supplementing on calcium, magnesium, zinc, chromium and other micro-minerals.

We know the problem, yet we keep promoting this type of practice once again, eating with no real thought about the detrimental consequences of these actions. Carbohydrates such as cakes, breads, cereals sweets and biscuits provide only empty calories with little or no nutrients. Natural sugar is a far better choice than added sugar disguised even in a "so called health or protein bar". Natural sugar can only be found in mother nature. The smallest and end-product of the macronutrient carbohydrate are Monosaccharides and like most nutrients are absorbed in the small intestine. It is usually the rate of transportation and absorption that is important here. Glucose and fructose are both quick to be absorbed but dependant on what nutrients you combine them with at the same time. A meal containing protein and fat decelerates the absorption rate than if they were eaten alone. Hence why fruit in its natural state is a better option than the juice of a fruit and having a few nuts or seeds with a boiled egg has always been a staple snack that I advise.

Drinking an apple juice or an orange juice sold in supermarkets is more, or less like having a can of coke. They contain so much more sugar and other additives and my advice is to stick well clear of them. The monosaccharides are an energy source; most of them provide about 4 Calories (kilocalories) per gram and burns quickly like paper on the fire with a desire for another hit! Sugar is one of the most addictive substances on the planet and is just has hard to give up as nicotine.

Some examples of food that contain a lot of free monosaccharides are fruits and fruit juices (glucose and fructose. Honey (glucose and fructose) lollies (glucose), syrups in the form of liquid glucose, corn syrup and invert sugar (glucose and fructose), fructose syrup, high fructose corn syrup, agave nectar and blackstrap molasses, are all high in fructose. Sweet white wine contains both glucose and fructose and having one drink per night, 365 days of the year, (thinking that this is fine) can lead to a weight gain of 7 kg per annum. Foods with added simple sugars include soft drinks, sports drinks, and energy drinks. Some of these energy drinks like '*Mother*' contain a particularly harmful contaminant aspartame, a biochemistry killer, creating hallucinations, excessive nervous energy, anxiety and irritability. Liquors, chocolate, sweetened dairy products and desserts contain mainly glucose. A well-known Australian Naturopath, Mona Hecke, specialising in children's health, revealed that midwives are telling young mothers 'to stay away from citrus fruit'. The rationale was that fruit is too high in sugar. The irony is that, it was ok to give a child Panadol (a drug) and synthetic milk powders yielding no nutritional value yet advised to stay away from real natural fruit as they contain far too much sugar! Fruit, as we already know has antioxidant properties, contains fibre, to assist bowel movements, supports immune system yet a Panadol dulls their nervous system and has no benefit what so ever! No wonder children are swollen, toxic, hyperactive and irritable ... they are stuffed to the brim, full of their own poop!

Magnesium, is by far the most important mineral for the breakdown of glucose and most of our western day population is deficient. Magnesium is responsible for about 700 chemical reactions in our body and is required to supply energy for all cells of the body, especially those of the nervous system. Magnesium plays a prominent role in glycogen synthesis and the metabolism of other sugar such as Galactose, fructose and mannose. Low magnesium levels can be found in people that have diabetes, pancreatitis and hypoglycaemia induced by a high refined carbohydrate diet. Potassium deficiency can also impair glucose metabolism. Thiazide diuretics cause a loss of both potassium and sodium in the urine, decreases glucose tolerance and can make diabetics worse.

To be fair to all, if you are having a problem with "carbs" and the negative effects, perhaps we need to ask the right question, do you have the availability of enzymes to help break down these molecules? We need to ask our self the question do we have too much carbs or are we not really using them to our advantage? We need a little carbohydrate to assist proteins assimilation that drives muscle growth in fact and neuro-synthesis of important hormones or chemical messengers that promote great emotional and mental health. The problem, too, along with food choice is that whilst your pancreas is busy shuttling off glucose to the cells, the other role of the pancreas, the release of digestive enzymes may be compromised. The pancreas produces these digestive enzymes which are naturally mixed with sodium bicarbonate, breaking down not only sugar but protein and fats and when this does not occur other problems may. Excessive exercise, aging, toxic exposure, and when the body's demand for enzymes exceeds the supply (fluctuating blood sugar levels), common health complaints may occur. Perhaps it may be the deficiency of digestive enzymes driving internal malabsorption and breakdown of carbs that is assisting the expanding waistline or our nutritional deficit? Take home message is that whole, unprocessed foods in general give rise to a lower glycaemic response, so eat small meals with some fruit, nuts and seeds and include easily digestible fats and proteins … A recipe for youth and a healthy Gut!

18

PROTEIN- A HIGHLY IMPRESSIVE AND VERY VERSATILE SUBSTRATE

Protein whilst synonymous with axe yielding muscle bound Vikings and Neanderthal looking males exploding out of, what looks like a size 6 kid's t-shirt, is an essential macro nutrient for survival beyond building muscle tissue alone. Protein became enormously popular in the 90s, thanks to Mr Atkins whom introduced "The Atkins Diet", a

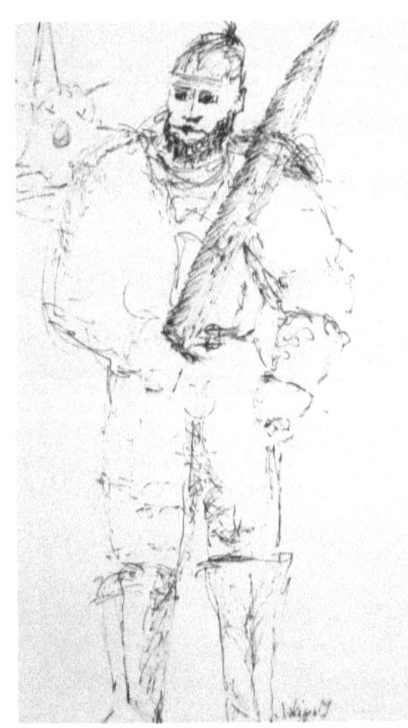

type of diet advocating high protein and high fat with little carbohydrates. Recently with the reintroduction of a similar diet called 'Paleo there has been an over emphasis on protein which has crowded out equally important substrates, lipids and carbs to our detriment!

Proteins, chemically are comprised of carbon, hydrogen and oxygen, like carbohydrates and lipids, however the difference is they also contain nitrogen atoms. Nitrogen are the links in the proteins and provide the name 'amino' to the amino acid. Proteins are more complex than the other substrates because of their structure. Put it this way, it would be like saying that all humans are the same, omitting the fact that we are culturally different. The Chinese differ from the Koreans, which are different from the Japanese, which are different again to the Vietnamese, yet all coming under the same umbrella of Asian. Unlike carbohydrates, that are composed of the same unit, glucose, which vary in length, protein means of prime importance and uses fragments of carbs and fats to perform bodily functions. They are vital working structures within all cells being versatile by nature. (33)

A protein is a long macro molecule that consists of approximately 20 different amino acids all joined together in different combinations with side groups attached. The protein in an egg is different to the protein in a piece of steak, which again is different to a plant-based protein found in a pea or a soya bean. Distinctive sequences determine the shape and the structure of proteins which also determine their role. As you would not expect a front row forward to squeeze into chimneys to do the role of a small chimney sweep, all proteins are not the same contain different structures and their functions are determined during protein synthesis. Animal flesh usually contain the 9 essential amino acids, histidine, isoleucine, lysine, leucine, methionine phenylamine, tryptophan, and valine. The difference between animal protein and vegetable proteins is that animal proteins contain all the essential amino acids whilst vegetable proteins do not, and for this reason animal proteins are primary proteins whilst vegetable proteins are secondary. These 9 essential amino acids cannot be manufactured by the body and must be obtained through food. Whilst some of the other 20 amino acids can be synthesised by the body, others must be obtained from the diet. If we are just eating rice, vegetables and fruit we can seriously compromise our protein requirement, even though these are high quality nutritious foods.

A hipster movement has adopted a similar diet to the 'Atkins' called 'Paleo'. This way of eating is not a new concept in which one completely avoids grains and all processed food (supposedly). Hmm, sounds like a plan. Whilst many health gurus advocate a "paleolithic diet, including the Australian "My kitchen rules" Chef Pete Evans as a modern way of eating, these guys forgot to mention that virtually all the protein our Palaeolithic ancestors ate were raw, including meat and eggs! The Paleo diet has been shown to surmount unwanted disorders that seems to be plaguing our western world, predominately it seems to fare well regarding health especially diabetes and obesity. What is unique and special about the Paleo diet is that it draws on an unusual *branch* of science, namely evolutionary theory. The Paleo diet is rooted in a much older tradition of what constitutes healthy living and proposes an aversion to modern day processing techniques. This way of eating has been around for more than thirty years. The statistics show that processed carbohydrates reign supreme. The real Paleo was introduced thousands of years ago, when stoves were not invented and, included meat freshly killed, raw and in season, not entirely omitting any food group ie grains. In any case, protein is primary, essential for survival and one of the most powerful anti-aging substrates with additional health benefits when consumed in a well-balanced diet. Whilst great in theory, according to one of Australia's leading nutritionist, Rosemary Stanton, we are not designed to eliminate a food group long term without negative consequences. (33) Ms Stanton also says, "thanks to fad diets like Paleo and sugar free, Aussies are ditching essential nutrients causing malnourishment- but we're also getting fatter". (35)

Whilst our digestive system prefers raw proteins, it is a necessity of cooking that reduces carcinogenic properties and harmful bacteria found in raw flesh. Heating though, will have an effect as proteins like lysine and cysteine can be destroyed, whilst glutamine is also sensitive to heat. Lysine is a Branch Chain Amino acid, (BCAA) required for growth and retards the growth of the herpes simplex 1 and 11 virus. Cysteine is one of the three amino acids of glutathione which plays a key role in deactivating the harmful "free radicals" that enter our body. It has been shown to reduce the toxicity of various liver toxins including pyrrolizidine alkaloids, (found in tobacco leaves), nitrosamine and acetaldehyde which builds up in the bloodstream of heavy alcohol consumers. Cysteine protects against toxic metals and chemicals and has one feature common with vitamin C, it promotes the absorption of iron from the small intestine. In the compound N-Acetyl -cysteine or NAC, it has been found to loosen mucous in the upper respiratory tracts and reduces the severity of the allergic contact dermatitis. It has been also shown to prevent the onset of peptic ulcers which have resulted from a combination of poor diet and the toxins stored in rice oil.

Glutamine is the precursor to the most abundant antioxidant in the body glutathione. (32) Since glutamine is a precursor of glutathione, and found in most animal flesh, eggs and vegetables, its supplementation in the clinical diet can be used to avoid oxidative stress damage. (31) It is a supplement that may be useful in the treatment of alcoholism, as it reduces the craving for alcohol. L-glutamine, is vital for preventing the translocation of microbes, supporting the digestive system after periods of physical stress when glutamine requirements are increased. It is involved in nitrogen transport and helps to maintain secretory igA, an immune marker functioning primarily by preventing the attachment of bacteria to the mucosal cells of the gut.

Methionine has been used to lower histamine levels in schizophrenics and in people that suffer from severe allergies. Together with inositol, and choline, it can be used for gall bladder and fatty liver conditions and cases of high cholesterol and triglycerides. Eggs contain all three ingredients and whilst the egg has been given an unfair trial over the years, due to its high cholesterol levels, the yolk contains these essential nutrients that power hair, nail and skin health.

Proteins can be metabolised and burned for energy or they can be important substrates which go on to form neurotransmitters and hormones in the body. They are important for the synthesis of our cellular enzymes, immunoglobulins and lipoproteins in cell membranes. So you see proteins in our foods are in fact the origin of many very important biochemical substances in our body. We can manipulate amino acid levels in the body through changing the composition of our daily diet and specifically by taking single amino acid supplements to gain some sort of therapeutic control over various clinical conditions that may arise throughout our life time. Having said that, we need to be aware that proteins in foods and some peptides, which are components of protein are frequently the cause of allergies because they may be absorbed into the body, cause inflammation or react with the gastrointestinal tract to cause problems such as gluten intolerance. Lectins and phytates are just some of those proteins found in beans and in fact most protein-based foods. Activated nuts is a result of people wanting to include this food group into their diet as a necessary form of protein however ingesting too much can cause GIT disturbances. Changing the natural structure of these foods in this instance has made them more bioavailable for people with a lectin intolerance thereby they can readily gobble their nuts without any complications to their GIT.

Are Protein supplements just pretend protein?

One of the interesting growth industries in health products has been the emergence of protein powders readily available to aid weight loss and build muscle mass. You may need them if you wish to build extra muscle or if you are devoid of protein in your diet, however we have become a society that over-uses protein. I think you get the message. Minority groups may require additional protein found in powder forms, particularly vegans, vegetarians or the elderly where the quality of protein intake is poor. All proteins are not the same. There are different levels of bioavailability and have various rates of release into the blood stream.

There are so many protein products containing synthetic anagrams of the real deal found naturally in food that can cause more internal drama than a Shakespearian play! The number of women that I counsel who struggle with their weight continually argue that their trainer insists that they have a protein shake as a meal replacement. The concept of taking a protein supplement is to address the loss of protein in their quest for weight loss. It does not help to lose weight. We are seeing more male looking females that are bottom-heavy with bulging upper bodies yet carry far too much fat deposited in areas where women do not necessarily want it (unless you are a Kim Kardashian copier). The question is do we really need protein in this false form and if so does the body recognise the compound as being a natural source of fuel?

Protein is the building block of our hair skin, nails and of course muscle. It is an essential macronutrient however many companies have taken advantage of this concept and introduced hundreds of different products designed to be anabolic. "At the end of the day" announced my chemistry lecturer in one of my first biochemistry sessions, whilst explaining the roles of macronutrients "all roads lead to fat". The fate of protein, if not required and used, is stored as, you guessed it, fat. Eating too much protein which is not being used in, i.e - expenditure, can increase weight, especially fat and therefore defeats the original purpose of gaining muscle or losing inches!

Because of the various primary, secondary and tertiary structures, the shape of the structure is quite important in protein biochemistry. In the same way that a right foot requires a right shoe the left foot requires a different one, the structure is critical to perform specific functions. Vegetarians and vegans are usually the ones that may fall in to the trap of this amino acid song and dance as whilst their choice may be based on ethics, their lack of skill in combining foods to address nutritional requirements have caused deficiencies and disorder. The quality of protein that we eat is determined by protein digestibility and its amino composition. Digestibility depends on the source and other foods eaten with it. Animal protein digestibility is between 90-99% whilst plant proteins are only about 70-90% and legumes and soy are about 90%. If one essential amino acid is missing, a cell must dismantle its own proteins to obtain it. The results may be obvious in appearance with acne, sagging skin, fatigue, loss of hair lustre, and less volume under the skin. (33)

Veganism and vegetarianism has become a very popular fad as while great in theory is not so good in the practical sense when it comes to our health. To ensure that you are getting the right combination of amino acids from the proteins in our foods use complimentary proteins like legumes that supply isoleucine and lysine with grains that contain methionine and tryptophan. Used together is a perfect combination to prevent deficiencies. Unless all of the essential amino acids are consumed, the body does not have all the necessary building blocks to construct the proteins that it specifically requires. Other vitamins and minerals become deficient too like B6, B9, B12, Iron and zinc, which are all energy providing nutrients. It is no wonder that this minority group suffer from fatigue and infertility. Alternatively, being an ovo-vegetarian that complements with eggs, the results can be a life changer! Eggs are naturally birthed from a chicken without being harmful to the chicken, especially when free range is chosen, there should be no moral dilemma.

Whey is from cheese manufacturing and when combined with strength training may increase protein synthesis only slightly. Advertising has shamelessly and unmistakeably advocated and promoted protein supplements to build huge swollen muscle development through social media platforms, trendy magazines and misinformed websites. The deamination or the stripping of the nitrogen from the amino acids places an extra burden on the kidneys to excrete the unused nitrogen. Deamination creates ammonia, which is then converted to urea, a less toxic compound which is then returned to the blood and filtered out in the urine. I once had a client who had placed herself on a disproportionately high protein diet for over 6 months. She lost an exorbitant amount of weight including muscle and fat. She came to me in a great deal of pain with red swollen marks that looked like severe burns covering most of her arms, torso and legs. To my horror, it looked like someone had thrown a house hold cleaner, 'Handy-Andy' over her, which is predominantly ammonia. Her liver and kidneys could not cope with the excess protein and had to deal with it accordingly and her body chose to use another excretory organ, the skin to eliminate the toxic load! Like many body builders preparing for competition and like other so-called magic solutions, these supplements may be more harmful long-term and do not necessarily provide the miracle that is originally sought out.

Digestibility.

Protein is the only substrate that is digested in the stomach. For proteins to be digested properly, down to its tiniest forms we need to have a significantly low pH, in other words the stomach need to be highly acidic between 2.8 -3. At the same time, the breakdown of protein also requires the action of a digestive enzyme, called pepsin which is released by the pancreas. After about 30 minutes to an hour the stomach squirts its contents in waves through to the duodenum, the entrance into the small intestine. The pancreas excretes two litres of alkalising bicarbonate into the duodenum every day activating the pancreatic enzymes that will further the protein digestive process in the small intestine. (33)

Whilst some people favour high protein diets for weight reduction it often leads to a continual craving for carbohydrate foods. Because we have starved the body of carbohydrates, the body uses the protein from structural and working proteins to create the energy or glucose. If there is an adequate supply of both fat and carbohydrates amino acids are spared and allowed to perform their functions.

Amino Acids (AAs) are also used to create other compounds called neurotransmitters. The amino acid, tyrosine is a precursor to Gabba, the chill out messenger, and both norepinephrine and epinephrine the flight or fight hormones. It also is used to make thyroxin, the metabolic rate regulator. Tryptophan found in chicken and turkey is a precursor to serotonin and melatonin, the sleep wake cycle neuro-modulator. To some extent, we can manipulate the levels of these neuro-hormones and neurotransmitter precursors by changing and or altering the balance of the substrates in our diet.

There is no question that a diet that supplies all the essential amino acids ensuring protein synthesis, comes from foods containing high quality proteins or the mix of complimentary proteins that contain the amino acids missing in the other. Whilst singling out amino acids too has become popular like lysine for Herpes and tryptophan in the treatment of depression, it is much safer to obtain these in protein rich foods, particularly with nutritious carbohydrates and fat to help facilitate their use. Once again, the synthetic supplements fall short in comparison to <u>mother nature</u>. More food for thought!!

<u>Functions of protein</u>

Type of Protein	Functions
Structural	Forms structural framework for various parts of the body, Examples: Collagen in bone and other connective tissues, and keratin in skin hair and fingernails
Regulatory	Function as hormones that regulate various physiological processes, control growth and development, as neurotransmitters, mediate reponses of the nervous system. Eg - Insulin regulates blood glucose level. Substance P which mediates sensation of Pain in the Nervous system

Contractile	Allow shortening of muscle cells, which produces movement. EG myosin and Actin
Immunological	Aids in responses that protect body against foreign substance and invading pathogens
Transport	Carry vital substances throughout the body EG Haemoglobin which transports most oxygen and some carbon dioxide in the blood.
Catalytic	Acts as enzymes that regulate biochemical reactions, EG salivary amylase, sucrose and ATPase

Table 1 consisting of function of protein

19

'OILS AIN'T OILS'

A long time ago, in my youth, a television commercial advertised a superior oil for the smooth and efficient running of automobiles. The claim was 'oils aint oils', and there is no doubt that these wise words still ring true. All oils are not the same and their difference is based on their chemical structure, whilst some can be damaging to our health, others have specific health benefits. I've said before that everything is based on chemistry and from a chemist's point of view, fats are made from carbons, oxygen and hydrogen. It is the point of attachment or where hydrogen bond in the chain of carbons that determine the point of saturation or not. Monounsaturated fat, poly unsaturated fat and saturated fats are not the same yet, all are required for great health. Cholesterol in itself is not the shady negligent character that we have been led to believe. Cholesterol is an important structural component of cells, hormonal function, vital for neurological

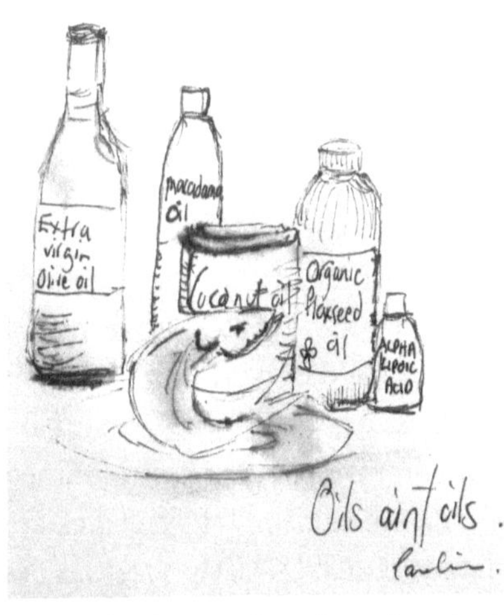

function and the number one body's repair substance in rebuilding tissues. If we lower functions of cholesterol by giving a cholesterol lowering drug we actually increase diseases like dementia, anxiety, depression, infertility, mineral deficiency, allergies and difficulty in healing.

For a long time now, we have been told to stay away from fat, but It is more likely the combination of tran's fat with processed foods that make us fat and lead to cardio vascular disease, pancreatitis, obesity, diabetes and some cancers. Deficiencies of fat may contribute to major hormonal issues so fat really plays a valuable role in both physical and mental health it is not fat that is the enemy actually, but sugar. Fats are a family known as 'the lipids'. Like your family the triglycerides-fats and oils is like your mother and father. The phospholipids are like your sisters, and the sterols, are your brothers. Each play a different role in the family, they are structurally unique whilst having the same basic units. (36)

Fats – which and what fat?

Generally speaking, fats and oils are naturally occurring complex mixtures of triacylglycerol molecules in which many different kinds of these molecules are present. The distinguishing fact between a fat and an oil is that fat is a mixture that is solid or semi solid at room temperature and generally obtained from animal sources. An oil, on the other hand is a liquid at room temperature and generally obtained from plant sources and from our cold-water fish. Triglycerides are the main constituents of natural fats and oils. (37) Triglycerides are the fats swimming around in our blood. Our cholesterol health is determined by the measurement of a combination of the triglycerides which are packaged in parcels, known as the high-density lipoproteins (HDLS) and the low-density lipoproteins (LDLS). The term good and bad cholesterol is really a myth, as both HDLS and LDLs are proteins acting as a transportation system delivering cholesterol throughout the body. As the same way a truck is used to cart and dump certain products, both HDL and LDL have a job to do and are equally important. The Low-density lipoproteins deliver the cholesterol in a capsule from the gut to the liver, then to the intestines, the blood and then to the tissues. The high-density lipoproteins take the old excess cholesterol and transports it back to the liver to be recycled, used as energy, excreted or to be stored as fat! The LDls present more of a health risk, as in excess is stored within the fat cells and accumulates in adipose tissue!

Cholesterol is a fat like substance called a sterol. Our body makes cholesterol from a molecule called Acetyl-co-A, derived from the dissemination of all the macro nutrients sugars, fats and proteins and approximately 80% is manufactured in our liver. The remainder of cholesterol comes from animal foods and some plant sterols, cholesterol is created from the fatty acids in these foods. Cholesterol is an essential part of our body, instrumental for hormone synthesis, sex hormones, adrenal hormones, vitamin D and bile salts. Vitamin D 3, helps you absorb calcium from the intestine and increases the amount of calcium in the blood. Another fat-soluble vitamin K 2, is necessary in this transportation system that drive the calcium to the bone and give bone flexibility. If there is too much calcium in the blood this may accumulate in the arteries and in the joints leading to inflammation and creating the stickiness within the lining of your blood vessels increasing blood pressure which then leads to CVDs.

Uncontrolled chronic inflammation, as already mentioned is the number one driver of most diseases specifically in this case; cardio vascular disease (CVDs), diabetes, male impotence, dementia, arthritis and other neurological disorders. It really may not be fat that drives cardio disorders, but the combination of excessive LDls, blood calcium levels, poor diet, toxin accumulation and arterial lining damage. If the endothelial lining of the arterial wall or tissue damage is created it swells making the gap smaller thereby increasing blood pressure. It is not necessarily cholesterol and plaque that drives CVDS but this chronic inflammatory process. We may have to rethink that caltrate or calcium tablet that your doctor has prescribed and switch to eating more greens. These provide an abundance of natural calcium recognised by the body for the body!

It is also important for skin protection, serotonin function (much needed to ward off depression and sleep deprivation). Cholesterol is the main fat for myelin sheath formation needed for concentration and memory. Cholesterol is also required for antioxidant transport like vitamin E and A and other enzymes (2)

We need fat and if we don't eat fat our body creates it, naturally. Some sterols are also derived from plants that have protective mechanisms. Common sterols are contained in vegetable, fruits nuts and seeds.

Sugars creates inflammation, not necessarily fat.

All cells and organs in the body require good blood flow for nourishment and to remove toxins generally for health that is why depletion is an important factor in our lifestyles which is generally missing. The number one driver of all the above is what we put into our mouth. Sugar. Sugar from excessive carbohydrates including alcohol, margarine and trans fats release inflammatory chemicals, called cytokines which contribute to Inflammation. Cholesterol only presents danger when it forms deposits on the arterial walls. When plaque breaks off and forms blockages, stops blood flow causing oxygen deficits, heart attacks and strokes. It is more likely that the constant damage to the lining of the arteries from genetically modified foods, and oils like safflower, canola and polyunsaturated fats increase this damage placing more pressure on the kidneys in order to keep the same volume of blood circulating around the body.

Phospholipids

Phospholipids are important constituents of cell membranes., They are both water and fat soluble thus enabling vitamins, hormones and other fat-soluble substance to pass easily in and out of cells and imperative for cognitive functioning. Sixty percent of our brain is made up of Omega three fats so when someone calls you a fat head, take that as a compliment! Fats, line the membranes that surround the cell, which is a bio-phospholipid layer. Too much saturated fat makes the cells hard and non-pliable. For nutrients to pass through this membrane we need to make sure that the fat surrounding all cells is penetrable, fluid and flexible so the movement of nutrients, minerals and vitamins can flow in and out of the cell as smoothly as possible. The body needs all the different types of fats, even the saturated fats, as they all play a different role from pregnancy, brain function, digestion, sports performance and down regulating inflammation. Eating fat does not make you fat and some fat promote weight loss being the best fat burning foods available. The *Ketogenic Diet,* is one of those diets that promote fat for this purpose and has been tried and tested on various athletes with positive outcomes. The Ketogenic *Diet* has also been used with great success in the treatment of metabolic conditions, such as cancer and epilepsy. This is by far one of the greatest diets to date that has had a pronounced effect on inhibition of these diseases however this is a subject for another book.

Omegas – balancing the equation is the key to healthy cholesterol levels.

Certain cultures have been termed 'disease free' from our modern-day diseases; such as obesity, heart disease and cancer. Further investigation took various researchers to study a small population that have been protected from these diseases. The Inuit of Alaska, have eaten primarily a high fat, moderate protein and very little carbohydrate diet, for centuries. Being hunter gatherers in nature and living in an extremely harsh environment, they feed off the fat from the land, mostly from seal meat and blubber. A diet rich in Omega 3 fats, full of essential minerals such as selenium and high amounts of Vitamins E, and vitamin D. These trace elements have somewhat disappeared in our western day diet and deficiencies in these vitamins have been associated with prostate cancer, ADHD and other neurological diseases. This diet has claimed to be anti-inflammatory and anti-cancerous. After numerous amounts of studies, the conclusion was that the ratio of Omega 3s and antioxidants ingested were responsible for inhibiting the modern-day diseases compared to current society's very high Omega 6 fatty diets.

Polyunsaturated fats can be divided into two categories, omega-6 and omega-3. Our diet is top heavy with omega-6 which has elevated disease states. Recent studies have expanded our understanding of the mechanisms by which Omega-3 Poly unsaturated fatty acids (PUFAs) may protect against hormonally driven cancers. The body cannot make these fatty acids and must obtain them from food sources or from supplements. Diets that are rich in fish oil has been known to lower stress and also retard depression. Three fatty acids compose the Omega-3 family: Alpha-linolenic acid, Eicosapentaenoic acid(EPA), and docosahexaenoic acid (DHA). Alpha-linolenic acid (ALA) is found in, some types of beans, and in flaxseed/linseed, and olive oils, unrefined whole grains, dark leafy greens, certain nuts, and seeds (mainly linseed, pumpkin seeds, walnuts, hempseeds and the oils extracted from them. The other two, (EPA) and (DHA), are found in cold water fish, including fish oil and supplements. EPA/DHA has been shown to inhibit angiogenesis.

The healthiest food sources of DHA and EPA are fish, especially cold-water species such as salmon, mackerel, anchovies, shellfish and sardines. The body can survive without seafood as the body has the capacity to synthesise EPA and DHA from alpha-linolenic acid (ALA). However, if we understand that the body converts only about 15% of dietary ALA to EPA and converts much less to DHA even in optimal conditions, fish is an ideal choice of omega-3. The process of converting ALA to EPA and DHA is hampered by many factors common to many of us in Australia. The dietary omega 6 fatty acids, dietary trans fatty acids, found in processed and fast foods and alcoholic beverages play a huge role in this disturbance of metabolism. When we eat cold water fish and supplement with fish oil, we are assured that we are getting the critical omega 3s in a way that allows our bodies to utilize them for our highest benefit.

At the end of the day, too much of anything is not always good. Fats only present danger when combined with certain sugars, which we have way too much. You have all probably felt the difference after the festive season where intake of high sugary laden foods and loads of champagne and beer flows, you may feel inflamed, swollen and fat. The amount of new years resolutions that involve giving up alcohol and starting an exercise plan is bigger than a Ben Hur production. Start low and go slow is the key as making grandiose plans may set you up for failure, as this is too hard to keep up with long term. Changes can be implemented in your diet and your lifestyle by modifying your intake and manipulating your diet by exchanging lesser quality fat for the better quality ones.

Type of lipid	Functions
Triglycerides (Fats and oils)	Protection, insulation energy storage
Phospholipids	Major lipid component of Cell membranes

Cholesterol-Sterols	Minor component of all animal cell membranes, precursor of bile salts, vitamin D and steroid hormones
Bile salts	Needed for digestion and absorption of dietary lipids
Vitamin D	Helps regulate calcium level in the body, needed for bone growth and repair
Adreno corticoid hormones	Helps regulate metabolism resistance to stress, salt and water balance
Sex Hormones	Stimulates reproductive functions and sexual characteristics
Eicosanoids Prostaglandins & leukotrienes	Have diverse effects on modifying responses to hormones blood clotting, inflammation, immunity, stomach acid secretion, airway diameter, lipid breakdown and smooth muscle contraction.
Other Lipids	
Fatty acids	Catabolised to generate adenosine triphosphate (ATP) or used to synthesize triglycerides & phospholipids
Carotenes	Needed for synthesis of vitamin A which is used to make visual pigments in the eyes. Also function as antioxidants.
Vitamin E	Promotes wound healing, prevents tissue scarring, contributes to the normal structure and function of the nervous system and functions as an antioxidant
Vitamin K	Required for synthesis of blood clotting proteins
Lipoproteins	Transport lipids in the blood, carry triglycerides and cholesterol to tissues and remove excess cholesterol from the blood

Table 2

20

ENZYMES: ARE THEY THE MISSING LINKS?

Rule of thumb, if food looks dead than it probably is. If the colour of that food is a sickly, yellowy brown the life has probably been cooked out of it and all that remains is a carcass, like a dead animal lying by the side of the road, fly blown and empty! The missing life component is probably 'enzymes'. Enzymes are substances that are produced by living organisms that act as an initiator to bring about biochemical reactions. In other words, Enzymes do things, and in all living cells, most of these catalysts are tertiary structured proteins, needed for the smooth biochemical reactions which occur spontaneously. These are the biomolecular machines that digest or break down all types of food and other molecules essential for maintaining great cellular health. When you eat, some enzymes, are used for the digestion of complex meals like amylase that break down carbohydrates, protease that break down proteins and lipase that digest fats. Some enzymes are responsible for fighting and engulfing dangerous microbes that enter our body whilst others are required to remove debris including broken down useless cells and toxins.

When I think back to my grandmother's day, if food didn't grow in the back yard, came from a chicken or a cow locally, swam in the river, or picked from a tree, we just did not eat it, nor was packaged food available. The only thing that came in on a truck shuttling down the boundary road was bottled milk, freshly baked bread, and the local daily rag, the local newspaper. I still remember the smell of lamb chops sizzling and hissing in a well-used pan, strangled by a cup of lard, on cold and frosty mornings. Cooking was simple. Hearty, solid old-fashioned stews, and meat and three types of vegetable. There was much cooking, baking and action in the kitchen and in contrast to this, the modern-day woman throws out the conventions of being tied to the kitchen and has been known to use the oven as a 'shoe cupboard'.

In the history of primates and the evolution of mankind, we as humans, are the only animals that cook food. Whilst the practice of cooking foods is common it destroys many of the enzymes and valuable nutrients in the foods, particularly some of the amino acids which make up the proteins. Since cooking changes the shape of these proteins, the heat denatures and inactivates them so that they do not work at all. Hence proteins are sensitive to increased temperature changes. Whilst there is a school of thought that pervades and states that cooking may be the cause of all humanities bodily illness, the thought of eating raw chicken flesh is disgusting. Raw chicken may be a possible breeding ground for campylobacter jejuni or salmonella, A nasty way to start your digestive tract on fire! Enzymes operate both chemically and biologically with science unable to measure or synthesize their biological or life energy. Biological force is the very core of every enzyme. In the maintenance of health and in healing, enzymes do the labour that drives metabolism. Almost all metabolic processes in the cell require enzymes to occur at rates fast enough to sustain life. The set of enzymes made in a cell controls which metabolic pathways occur in that cell and the greatest source of digestive enzymes are contained in raw foods whilst refined and processed food are negligent.

Enzymes are created by our organs and glands through a sophisticated internal telecommunication system. These enzymes are custom designed and specific to perform a vital role. Enzymes possess a life force, giving off electrical energy as they work. They are so much more than just the mechanical nature of being a catalyst as a catalyst is a compound which speeds up or assists these chemical reactions. Pepsin, secreted from the stomach catalyses proteins such as meat and eggs in the digestive process, amylase breaks down sugars, lactase breaks down dairy products etc. The pancreas releases many digestive enzymes to catabolise foods. If you have pancreatic cancer these enzymes are faulty. Supportive enzymes like digestive enzymes are usually administered so that nutrients will be assimilated and used properly.

I have often suggested having fresh pineapple pieces 15 minutes before meals as the bromelain has anti-inflammatory properties and enzymatic in nature helping your food to break down. Papain from paw-paw can be beneficial too. Although not customary in our culture, for centuries the Japanese have not been afflicted with our modern-day diseases as they typically have salads first, followed by sashimi and then beef. I have a Japanese friend that dines on 4 course meals most nights yet has the most amazing blood work. Whilst he has been prescribed lithium for his mental health, he swims every day with bouts of resistance training. He manages his disorder with eating like a king and training like a champion and whilst he is over sixty years of age, has the blood work that resembles a 35-year-old. It is a good habit to have a colourful salad, loaded with enzymes and nutrients combined with an easily digestive piece of oily fish, steak or chicken at least twice per week. Stir-fry's are a great nutritional option as it is a mix of cooked, easily digestible proteins with some essential fats in the form of omega 3s. Lignin's in the form of flaxseeds sprinkled over salad or vegetables is a natural source of omega 3 adding bulk to salads and known to assist in fat loss. Eating a rainbow every day, bright and colourful food are full of wonderful life enhancing properties.

21

NOT SEEING THE FOREST THROUGH THE TREES.

"The ultimate measure of a man is not where he stands in moments of comfort and convenience, but where he stands at time of challenges and controversy".

Martin Luther King

I learned at an early stage of my nutritional career that it is far easier to prescribe a pill than to change a lifestyle. Working, alongside a nutritional biochemist, I asked him, why after having a successful natural practice he should build a nutraceutical company. He stated that Unfortunately after many years of being a practitioner, he had also learned the hard way. People expect instant results with little or no work from themselves. My heart sank. I had recently graduated

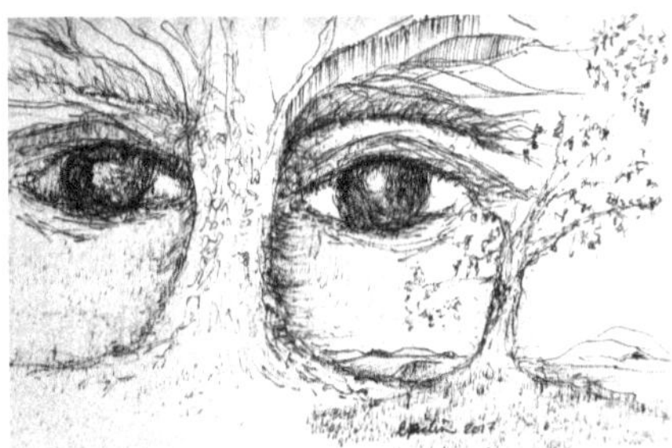

and had possessed grandiose intentions of changing the world with my new-found knowledge. My goal then became apparent and I knew more than ever that I was up for the challenge! And now, from my own experience, I believe that most people are in search of that single, wonder pill to fix them. One pill to address all your needs? Not possible! I still shake my head in disbelief as day in and day out, it seems that most people still do not 'get it'.

When should one's accountability in health matters cease? Handing over our power to the medical authorities, in many cases will end up hastening our demise. Band aid medicine like taking thyroxine, ant-acids, blood pressure lowering, anti-cholesterol drugs will not help us in the long run. Get to the source of your problem. Why are you over eating? Why is your metabolism sluggish? Why are you hypertensive? Why do you have acne? The questions 'why' is more paramount than ever. Why, is finding out the reasons for doing the 'what you do'. Once you know this you then can determine self-regulating habits in a quest for overall health if this is important to you.

I cannot help wondering if there really is an association between how we think and therefore how we act that contributes to the disease continuum. If this is so, then all disorders may be undeniably a result of the relationships between the physical, the spiritual and the emotional. Even a cough can be associated with a nervous predisposition. A single thought can alter your mood and effect your whole day. How often do you think of something negative and when it happens you tell yourself "I told you so"! The thought creates the energy for that 'something' to occur. If this can be done to induce a negative response or reaction, then surely it can be used to create a positive one.

You only have one body and your reality is not a fantasy. You are the only one that can truly answer the question, have I been kind to myself or have I been respecting my body? This book is not designed to aggravate, incite fear or to antagonise you, but if it does then I have stirred something within you. This is a book to be used as a resource to remind you that you have the power to correct minor dysfunctions before they escalate to the point where they are out of control. We have an abundance of great food books with enticing and easy to prepare recipes to be taken advantage of. Recreational centres and gyms that exist on practically every street corner, to fill the entire world over-and-over again so then we have to ask ourselves "why are we not using them"? or "why are we in such a mess in the first place"? Actions speak louder than words and whilst most of us 'know so much' it is only action that has the power. Put down the fork and walk is the basis of restorative health in eliminating the junk from your trunk. This simple act will place us all in good stead for a stress-less and healthier life.

If our life is about management and each day is significant, taking on a consciousness that places you in the here and now regardless of having any disease is the only way to live life. Depression is associated with living in the past and anxiety is really a fear of the future. If you live in the here and now and in this very moment, there can be none of these. The power of the mind should never be underestimated. It is incredible that even if we have been granted the affliction of a debilitating disease, we too can live a full and productive life, bereft of symptoms. It is all about management. This may sound precocious or dismissive but what if it is easy as this? *Easier said than done*", you might say, or "It's alright for you, as you do not have it", point taken, but trust me we all live with some affliction or another and shit does happen. This is a fact. It is also our perception of the circumstances of our life that can encourage disorders and disease. I do know this though, if we do not address any issues of concern in their early stages then don't be too surprised when you too get on that disease fight or flight ship

Life is about movement and the transfer of energy. Seasons change, tides ebb and flow, the moon and stars appearing on the night horizon, day changes into night and so on and so forth. Change is happening before our very eyes, yet whilst these changes occur we stand still in our own minds. We are more likely to change our hair colour, geographical location, and car, yet the biggest change must come from within to create the 'without'!!! Without the disease, without the weight, without the drama or without the problems. As we age, changes are harder than ever, as even if there is a wish and a will for a positive outcome, we may wait for our insecurities and self-doubt to dissolve. Trust me, I am the biggest coward ever and change is difficult. Yet, if one doesn't move and does nothing, nothing will move, and nothing will change. To move from pain to pleasure is by far the greatest motivation however sometimes the pain that we experience is what we know and ironically, where we find comfort. But If we could only see ourselves five years, or ten years from now, then may be that image may facilitate change. It may be the initiation, to move and to make positive contributions toward the life that we could lead, away from the one that we are now living. It must start somewhere. The feeling of lacking, fear, self-doubt and insecurity arise from the dark force inside of us, the monster within. These feelings contribute to the blocks that keep us where we are, may be fat, may be nearly finished and may be at a major turning point in our life, Fifty!.

What you do as a living does not define you but what you do in living can. Just like the trip in the BMW, if you are unprepared and unaware, be prepared for accidents. A lifetime of bad habits can accumulate and over time it takes its toll but the one thing that is apparent, is energy given equates to energy provided. Disease thrives in an acidic host and feeds primarily on sugar. Never under estimate the power of nutrition, your thought process and the role of emotional stress, all instrumental in the development of disease and the ultimate disease, cancer. Nutrition and the lack thereof is paramount to health, it provides the foundation. It sets the stage for your whole life.

Great health these days is not by default, it is a choice. To blame another person for your health conditions is ludicrous as you are the solo commander of your body, your ship. Any thinking person has no excuse as knowledge is power, yet knowledge is not true power unless it is practiced! You are the pilot and you control or manage how you think and feel. Be careful of your thoughts, as they become your words, and naturally, actions will follow. By default, you set the stage for each day and as <u>contrary</u> as this may sound, just like the pilot in a helicopter that hands over the control. Before he lets go, and firmly places that instrument in your hand, you are the one that reassures him that you have 'got this'. Be careful what you read and be careful of what you place in your mouth, become the critical thinker and ask the question 'why'? Asking questions gives you greater understanding, and acceptance so you can act from a love-based state and not from fear to change your direction for the better. Put knowledge into real wisdom.

One life, your life … and your life ultimately is up to you!

REFERENCES

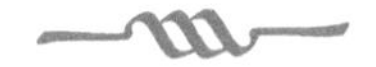

1   www.who.int/whr/2001/media_centre; who - mental disorders affect one in four people. The world health organisation.

2   Smith, Clark; Postmodern wine making; rethinking the modern science of an ancient craft. California press; 2 Nov 2013

3   Oseiki,H; Cancer; the importance of clinical Nutrition in prevention and treatment.

4   Vander Kraats, B.A, N.D dip acup, B.D.M How to have younger arteries and prevent heart disease and strokes

5   Tzu, Sun; The art of war

6   Duke, James; Anti-aging prescriptions.

    Is our modern-day diet killing us?

7   Statham, Bill; The chemical maize.

The village

8   Pinker, Susan; The village effect ;how face to face contact can make us happier and healthier

9   Robert Waldinger; What makes a good life? Lessons from the longest study on happiness.

10   https://www.theguardian.com/technology/2017/nov/09/facebook-sean-parker-vulnerability-brain-psychology.

Trust your gut

11   https://www.collinsdictionary.com/dictionary/english/instinct

12   https://chriskresser.com/9-steps-to-perfect-health-5-heal-your-gut

13   Yeasts in the Gut: From Commensals to Infectious Agents; Jürgen Schulze, PD Dr. rer. nat. habil.[*,1] and Ulrich Sonnenborn, Dr. rer. nat.[2] Dtsch Arztebl Int. 2009 Dec; 106(51-52): 837–842. Published online 2009 Dec 1. doi: 10.3238/arztebl.2009.0837

14   http://juicing-for-health.com/4rs-to-restoring-your-gut-health

15   Zonulin & Leaky Gut: A discovery that changed the way we view inflammation, autoimmune disease and cancer!

     http://primaldocs.com/members-blog/zonulin-leaky-gut

16   Maroof H[1], Hassan ZM, Mobarez AM, Mohamadabadi MA Lactobacillus acidophilus could modulate the immune response against breast cancer in murine model. J Clin Immunol. 2012 Dec;32(6):1353-9. doi: 10.1007/s10875-012-9708-x. Epub 2012 Jun 19.

17   http://www.ncbi.nlm.nih.gov/pubmed/22711009

Water is it the forgotten macronutrient

18   Water, Hydration and Health Barry M. Popkin, Kristen E. D'Anci, and Irwin H. Rosenberg Nutr Rev. Author manuscript; available in PMC 2011 Aug 1. Published in final edited form as: Nutr Rev. 2010 Aug; 68(8): 439–458. doi: 10.1111/j.1753-4887.2010.00304.x

19   Edwards 'Sir peter and Lady Patricia; Glow with health; a healthy liveable, nutrition plan for the whole family. Pan harmony international 2002

20   Benton D., Burgess N. The effect of the consumption of water on the memory and attention of children.Appetite. 2009; 53:143–146. [PubMed

21   H.H. Mitchell Journal of Biological Chemistry 158, Dec 2, 2016

22   Elaine Magee, MPH, RD 19 easy ways to get your 9 servings a day. *Web;MD Weight Loss Clinic*

Reviewed By Brunilda Nazario, MD; *http://www.medicinenet. com/script/main/art.asp?articlekey=55983*

23   Kuiper GG, Carlsson B, Grandien K, et al. Comparison of the ligand binding specificity and transcript tissue distribution of estrogen receptors alpha and beta. *Endocrinology* 1997; 138:863–870. [PubMed]

24   http://www.breastcancer.org/risk/factors/plastic

25   Mol Cancer Ther. 2002 May;1(7):515-24. The xenoestrogen bisphenol A induces inappropriate androgen receptor activation and mitogenesis in prostatic adenocarcinoma cells. Wetherill YB[1], Petre CE, Monk KR, Puga A, Knudsen KE

26   www.betterhealth.vic.gov.au

27   http://foodandspirit.com/about/dr-deanna-minich Functional Nutritionist, Author, Artist, Yoga Practitioner 3

Has the Dairy been taken from our dairy?

28   mercola.com/sites/articles/archive/2009/07/09/the-devil-in-the-milk.aspx

29   https://www.foodsense.

30   dranthoygustin.com What is betohydroxybutrate . (article) www.perfectketo.com 2015

31   .ww.ncbi.nih.gov/pubmed/10356308 "Molecular genetics and metabolism."1999 Jun;67(2):100-5. Glutamine, as a precursor of glutathione, and oxidative stress. Amores-Sánchez MI[1], Medina MA

32   Buist, Robert A. BSc (Hons), PhD, A.R.A.C.I Nutritional biochemistry of proteins; postgraduate course in clinical nutrition

33   Whitney, Elllie; Rolfes, Sharon Rady; Crowe, Tim; Cameron Smith, David; Walsh, Adam; Understanding Nutrition; Australian and New Zealand edition 2011

34   http://www.smh.com.au/lifestyle/diet-and-fitness/nutritionists-warn-of-dangers-in-paleo-dieting-20140805-100iup.html

3 5   www.news.com.au/lifestyle/.../diet/... diets.../78bb62db8385df48a565fe7f8a79a88b- May 11 2016

36   Glutathione Metabolism and Its Implications for Health[1]

Guoyao Wu[2], Yun-Zhong Fang[*], Sheng Yang[†], Joanne R. Lupton, and Nancy D. Turner

37   Whitney, Elllie; Rolfes, Sharon Rady; Crowe, Tim; Cameron Smith, David; Walsh, Adam; Understanding Nutrition; Australian and New Zealand edition 2011

38   Stoker, Stephen.H;General, organic and biological chemistry. Fifth edition